FUNdamentals™ of Outstanding Dental Teams

Vicki McManus, RDH

Foreword by Anthony Robbins

Other contributors: A. Paul Bass, III, Nate Booth,
Linda Drevenstedt, Carol Hacker,
Paul Homoly, Dyan Hunter, Cathy Jameson,
Brenda Kaesler, Linda Miles, Penny Reed,
Alan & Sandy Richardson, Doug Smart

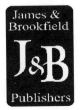

James &
Brookfield
J&B
Publishers

FUNdamentals™ of Outstanding Dental Teams
compiled by Vicki McManus

Cover Design:	PAULA CHANCE
Editing:	KATHY MEYER
Book Layout:	DARLENE NICHOLAS
PHOTOGRAPHY:	KEVIN MCMANUS

For more information, contact:
James & Brookfield Publishers
P.O. Box 768024
Roswell, GA 30076
(770) 587-9784

Library of Congress Catalog Number 97-076406

ISBN: 0-9658893-0-0

10 9 8 7 6 5 4 3 2 1

Dedication

To my supportive husband, Kevin, and
our wonderful children, Hillary and Sean.

Special thanks to our Team

Anthony Robbins — for his message, model, and motivation.
Each contributor and featured writer — for their
dedication to this project.
James & Brookfield Publishers and their creative
and editorial design team.
My coach — Sharron McLeod.
My mentors — John Brantley and Stephen Moroski.
Mike & Vicki Egan and the network of coaches
with Fortune Practice Management®.
William Mays of the National Dental Network.
Susan Love, Sharon Sperling, Gene & Yvonne Dinkins,
Albert & Dorsel McManus, and so many others
that are a part of my personal and professional team.

Table of Contents

☺ v

Foreword

If there is one thing that I could tell you that will change your life make you money and create fulfillment, it would be to **become a team player**. You are already a part of a team, but are you a team player?

I don't care how big your practice is, how many people you contribute to, how much money you make, if you are not continuously growing, you are not happy.

As Ray Kroc would say, "When you're green you grow, when you're ripe you rot." Wouldn't you agree that the times you are happiest in life are when you are challenged and growing inside?

Most of us are trapped in a relationship with our comfort zone. We have levels and expectations for our relationships and our practices where we are comfortable. If we remain in our comfort zone too long, we get in a place where we have no purpose for expanding and begin to turn to things outside ourselves — food, alcohol, drugs, or other substances — to try to stuff down the emotions we have inside.

As human beings, we will do more for those we care about than we will ever do for ourselves. It's not money or acknowledgment that counts. There comes a point in time where most of us have more than we need. This is especially true in the wealthiest country on earth! What I have found to be the primary, long-term human motivator is the ability to contribute to others in a meaningful way.

That is why you surround yourself with a team. So that you have people around you who will push you to contribute. You will do more to support your coworkers, your patients, and your family than you will ever do for yourself. This book is about making sure your team members challenge you to expand and grow on a daily basis.

As cofounder of Fortune Practice Management®, I am excited to see the impact we are having on healthcare teams. Vicki has done an excellent job creating a team of dedicated professionals to bring you the teambuilding technology in this book. By utilizing the talents of people from within our organization, as well as other known professionals in the field, she has created a resource for you to refer to again and again. The diversity of voices combines to share with you *the principles of team* that will impact your relationships with your professional team, as well as your personal team. FUNdamentals™ of Outstanding Dental Teams will guide your journey of connecting with those around you in a way that is fun, innovative, and precisely designed to give you the basic tools of team development. I invite you to actively participate while you read to maximize the impact on your team.

Don't let your team wait another day to claim the happiness you deserve. As you move toward creating your vision and the team of your dreams, remember to ***love the moment, not just the future***.

Anthony Robbins

Introduction
FUN: our Gift to Dentistry

Vicki McManus, RDH

It's 6:00 a.m. Bzzzzzz. The alarm sounds the arrival of a bright new day. You bound out of bed anticipating getting to the office, scrubbing up and setting the drills a blazing! After all, your patients love you, your staff worships you, and your suppliers jump at your beck and call. Overhead is under control, no one has asked for a raise in eight months, and all your patients pay for their treatment at time of service. Life is a dream.

Actually, this scenario is a dream for most dentists. Faced with rising overhead, demanding staff, and budget considerations from patients — not to mention technology that has gone into hyperdrive — most dentists and their teams are feeling overwhelmed in this age of information. At a time when communication is more critical than ever, we seem to be having more challenges than ever in this area of our lives.

FUNdamentals™ of Outstanding Dental Teams will improve communication on your team, and it will enhance every aspect of your practice! Here's the FUNdamental™ Strategy overview:

Focus is on shared vision, agreements, goals.
Understanding each person's values, rules, and motivation.
Never-ending improvement in systems, relationships, and technology.

The team building process is both dynamic and interactive. Creativity, flexibility, relationships, and communication styles come together to create a quality environment for both patients and staff. Traditionally, dental teams do not receive much cross-function training. Hygienists and clinical assistants rarely understand the duties of the business office. The business administrators possess limited clinical knowledge, and only the doctor monitors the financial health of the business. Dentistry too often operates in a compartmentalized fashion that grossly underutilizes the talents paid for; employees are expected to show up, work, and leave. Understanding how they support the structure of the business has not been deemed necessary, when in fact it is *vital* to the health of the practice!

Why focus on developing an outstanding dental team? The answer is simple: to raise the standard of patient care and to reap the emotional and financial rewards so richly earned – and deserved – as healthcare provider. This is readily accomplished by creating what Dr. Paul Homoly describes as "team harmony." Top performance teams share some not so surprising qualities:

1. Staff shares psychological ownership of the practice.
2. Creativity and agility abound, providing a competitive edge.
3. Everyone understands "interdependence" and their role.
4. Financial incentives beyond traditional salary and benefits exist.
5. There is stability in workforce, decrease in turnover.
6. They effectively utilize each team member's skills.
7. Never-ending improvement of systems, technology and relationship exists.

Think of teams as an anthill. Worker ants gather food and build. The drones are responsible for serving the queen. And, of course, the queen works feverishly to insure the viability of the colony. Assuming ants could speak, could you imagine one worker ant turning to another and saying, *"I'm working really hard so that one day I can become a queen. If there is anything that I can do for you, please let me know. I believe that if I can support other ants in my community, then we can all enjoy a better work environment."* Maybe I have a bigger imagination than some, but even I would find it hard to believe such a thought crossing the mind of an ant. There is only one time when ants would consider stepping outside their boundaries to assist others in the colony — when they are faced with crisis and the hill is threatened.

Ants represent traditional teamwork. Each member is assigned tasks based on expertise in a particular area. When there is a crisis, such as a labor shortage or need to condense the schedule, everyone pitches in to help out. This is the old model of dentistry. Assistants, hygienists, and business administrators interact to exchange vital information pertaining to patient care. Each knew only the rudimentary skills required to function in other departments. The good news is that this is changing within dentistry.

What's needed is a new model that reflects synergy and increased information flow throughout the team; a team model that encourages cross-training, flexibility, and results. I call this the **Connected Team Model.**

We have all become familiar with computer technology and have an appreciation for the capabilities of a PC. Many offices are also discovering the advantage of having multiple terminals that utilize a networked design system, common language, data, and format. These practices boost bottom line profits, serve the patients at a higher level, and decrease the workload by decentralizing information. Tasks that once took many man-hours and elaborate systems to track can now be handled with one or two keystrokes!

What does this have to do with creating a connected team? Everything! Ask yourself these questions. Was the group of people that I currently work with brought together by design or by circumstance? *(network design)* Do we have policies, agreements, and training in place that allows each person's knowledge to be integrated in our "pool of knowledge?" *(common language and data)* Do we have planned weekly staff meetings that allow us time to continually integrate our principles of quality patient care and outstanding team performance? *(common format)*

As a consultant, I have observed that many dental teams have been formed out of haphazard necessity and not out of effective design. When a doctor first begins, he/she can establish a private practice and hire staff — without knowledge or experience in doing so — and work diligently to build the patient base, adding staff as the practice grows. Another option is to purchase an existing practice with staff in place and the doctor then shapes his or her style into the current patterns of the practice. Each staff member brings some knowledge and background to the team, and very little training is in place to integrate new people into the culture of the team. If cooperation is achieved with staff, it is by sheer accident and the team doesn't know how to repeat this success. Is this sounding familiar?

As you can see, the primary difference between a "team" and a "connected team" is the degree of integration of a common purpose, language and operating principles. This book will explore how we achieve what Anthony Robbins describes as C.A.N.I.!® (Constant And Never-ending Improvement)[1] in the area of networking our potential. The success strategies of the 80's and 90's will not work in the new century. Just as the computer industry moved from mainframe to PC, DOS to Windows, isolated to Internet, we must continue to shape our destiny by shaping our teams. Creating team ownership and a sense of interdependence will provide your practice with the creativity and agility needed to prosper in the years to come. Practicing the FUNdamentals in this book will propel your team to solid success!

[1] C.A.N.I.!® (Constant And Never-ending Improvement) is a registered trademark of the Anthony Robbins Company.

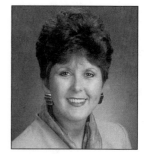

Chapter One

'Model' the Best:
The Dentist as Team Leader

Linda Miles, CSP, CMC

The greatest mistake you can make in life is to be continually fearing that you will make one. — ELBERT HUBBARD

In order for a piece of machinery to work effectively, all parts must be in sync. A dental team functions the same way. Each member of the team has a distinct purpose in the day-to-day operations. In order for patients to be served in the best possible environment (the purpose for each day), each member must be in sync. The dentist (leader) of the team must call the shots and be the role model of dedication to the daily outcome.

The fuel feeding the engine is a blend of respect, recognition, and shared rewards. Vision and commitment to that vision are realized only when the team members are aware of everyone's equal value.

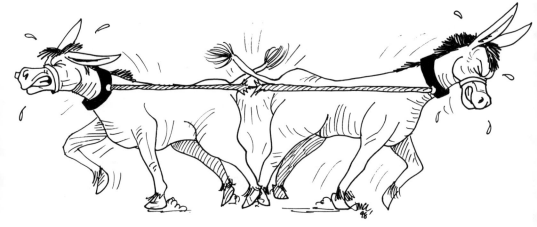

ARE YOU HEADING IN THE SAME DIRECTION?

When I ask dentists their most frustrating aspect of practicing dentistry, the response is always the same — *staff relations.* From Virginia to California, every practice that I work with faces the same issues of team building.

For twenty years I have spoken to this challenge and my message remains clear. Hire the best, contribute to their training, and care for them as family. What I'd like to share with you are some distinctions of a team-based practice and how the dentist becomes the leader of this team. As you will discover in this book, there is a vast difference between cohesive groups, teams, and top performance teams. We will show you ways to connect your team members to create results beyond your expectations.

Individuality within teamwork is a plus if the parts of the team respect the others' strengths and accept their weaknesses. Seeing something that needs to be done and doing it without being asked or told (initiative) is part of teamwork. The dentist/leader must be willing to delegate while at the same time demonstrating that he or she is willing to do whatever it takes to get the job done. Strong team leaders are ready and willing to be the missing link if the need arises.

There are two basic leadership styles that one can display. The first is the autocratic/dictatorial style. This is best described as the "My way or the highway" or the "Do as I say, not as I do." This style offers absolutely no benefit. In fact, it creates an unsafe environment of fear and low self-esteem, often resulting in staff turnover. This is in part because the "rigid ruler" spends time evaluating the dynamics of the day to determine how the tomorrows of the world can be designed without a glitch. These unrealistic expectations create work environments not conducive to teamwork. Whenever there are unexpected changes in scheduling, challenges in collections, or decreases in new patient flow, the staff follows the example of the doctor. They begin to lay blame, defend, and justify their actions, without considering how they could work together to create a solution to the challenges. Their priorities are: how do I save my skin, avoid the next round of "constructive" criticism, and make it through another day? They have very little emotional energy left to focus on quality patient care or the health of the business. Is it a wonder that patient retention is also a major challenge for these practices?

The second type of leadership is participatory, whereby the dentist becomes the leader of a team working toward a common purpose. The overall quality of work produced, care given, and rewards received are higher; as is staff and patient retention. Participatory team management allows all members a voice in decisions that directly affect them. This dramatically translates into creativity and self-esteem of each staff member, treatment and care for your patients, and more dollars at the bottom line of your profit statement.

Participatory leadership demands a certain philosophy as well as a style of leadership. Making such a shift involves a conscious choice to eliminate current thought processes and replace them with others. Working merely on changing the practice's surface behavior increases fatigue and frustration, and the temptation is to revert to old styles when faced with challenges. Be sure to explain this philosophical shift to your staff and request their support. To learn more about paradigm shifts, I recommend you read <u>The Seven Habits of Highly Effective People</u> by Steven Covey. Once you have internalized this paradigm shift, then it is easier to make the necessary changes in behavior.

In situations where the dentist is a more passive person, stronger team members can claim too much independence and authority, thus, undermining the whole team. The ideal balance of decision-making power is 51% dentist/owner and 49% total team. The doctor always has the final vote which he/she uses scrupulously.

To become a true team with participatory management, you must first understand that this style of leadership is a process of creating team 'work.' It is not an instant solution, nor a quick fix to all your problems. The ongoing nature of this process is consistently motivated by first becoming motivated yourself. Let's take a moment to discover the characteristics of a "team" dentist as a leader.

He or she has:

Loyalty — to the mission/vision, patients, and practice goals.
Enthusiasm — for dentistry and life. Can't expect the staff to be if you are not.
Attitude — always consistently positive.
Diversity — accept the differences in staffs' and patients' personalities, age, work ethic, and culture.
Enjoyment — in daily tasks and in life in general.

Respect, Responsibility, Rewards, Recognition — 4 R's of
   motivation.
Stick-to-it-tive-ness — consistency.
Health — we can't sell health if we don't have it.
Integrity — ability to walk the talk, live the rules.

Knowing the daily priorities of the team is essential to cohesiveness.
All members of the dental team must put the patient first, the practice as
a healthy business second, and their own needs and wants last. Create
job descriptions and daily tasks for each position that reinforce these
priorities. This foundation of accountability fosters high-level support.

Another way to create staff accountability is to monitor the
progress of the practice on a daily, weekly, and monthly basis. Each
person or department gives personal progress reports on their
particular part of the practice — operative, hygiene, and business
administration. The owner must share the financial standing of the
practice, with the exception of individual salary levels and doctors'
compensation, with his/her staff and allow for their participation. In
this partnership, the staff is more inclined to think of the health and
profitability of the business, rather than personal agendas, creating
and nurturing an atmosphere of trust.

Meanwhile, here's an effective way to address the challenge of the
non-participation of a team member, someone who is pulling against
the vision of the practice. You must confront them. You must let them
know it is obvious and they are on a 30-day notice to make changes.
Offer support and discuss specific ways that they can change their
attitude, behavior or performance. If they feel it is too much, then
their letter of resignation will gladly be accepted within 30 days.
Confronting nonperformance becomes easier as the doctor/owner sees
the improvement in office enthusiasm from the remaining committed
staff members after each successful confrontation.

As team leaders, dentists must insure constant growth and
improvement. They must clarify their vision and convey it in a way
that is ultimately shared by each team member. The doctor projects
this vision five years into the future. At each planning session, drop
the current year and pick up one-year into the future. Stagnation and
burnout occur when the energy of the shared vision becomes dim.
Without annual reestablishment of goals that stretch our abilities

and expand our vision, the practice slides downhill. The practice is either growing or shrinking. There is no in-between.

With growth and progress comes occasional failure. In fact, the most successful people of our time, whether in the sports arena, scientific research, or innovators are wrong most of the time. Babe Ruth is noted for having made the most home runs during his time. Did you realize that he also held the record for the most strikeouts? Thomas Edison successfully invented the light bulb after 9,999 separate experiments. As a coach for your team, you must learn to see "mistakes" as learning experiences and a positive part of innovation. Let me clarify: when a mistake is made it is tolerated *the first time*. Repeatedly making the same mistake indicates a flaw in the system, training, or ability of that person to complete a task. Analyze and review the situation with the person to determine where the breakdown is occurring. Create ways to monitor the process and evaluate as needed until the final positive outcome is achieved.

By tolerating innovative mistakes, we encourage creativity in the practice. I believe that the dental environment should be fun, invigorating, stimulating, and exciting. In a practice where creativity, vision, and purpose are in place, this is the environment. As the coach of the team, the doctor must be willing not to have all the answers. That's right, you must be willing NOT to have the answers to the challenges facing the team. Rely on the team to mastermind solutions according to the practice's vision, boundaries, and expectations.

The one aspect of team leadership that falls out of place most frequently is consistency. Once you have set the standards, you must become self-disciplined and hold every team member accountable for their role, not letting emotions or frustrations cloud your leadership. Old habits are hard to break. As you gain strength as a leader, it may be helpful to think of these new found strengths as muscles. We all know that if we go to the gym and work out for a period of time, we can get our bodies in great shape. Have you ever noticed how quickly we lose that shape once we stop working out? The same is true for leadership and coaching skills. As you invest in your staff, invest in yourself as well. Attend courses with your staff. Partner with a coach for in-office training and ongoing coaching of the practice. We all, even the team leader, need someone to hold us accountable.

Leadership is about balance in both your personal and professional lives. In your professional life there are three arenas that must be mastered equally well to maintain balance. You must have savvy business acumen, strong clinical and technical skills, and excellent people skills. Without each of these elements in place, you will miss out on the long-term emotional and financial rewards of your career.

The dentist can delegate the management responsibilities of the practice. However, he/she must still show up as the leader. No one is going to have as much care or concern for your business as you will. As you delegate responsibility, ensure that there are checks and balances in place so that you are always informed of decisions that impact the practice. As a leader, it is your responsibility to schedule time to meet with key people in the practice to review the business plan and make adjustments where necessary to ensure long-term success.

As a clinician, the dentist must be the role model for comprehensive care. The staff will fall in line with the doctor's philosophies — make sure you reinforce your beliefs on a regular basis. Stay in tune with the latest in clinical excellence through courses, audio tape series, and professional journals. Dentistry seems to be changing at the speed of light, don't get caught in the dark!

As a coach, you must develop people skills to guide your team. It is no longer acceptable to say "That's just the way I am. It's my personality to be short, direct or abrupt with others. People can take me or leave me." Believe me. They will leave you. Our marketplace is dictating that we provide a higher quality service with lower cost and friendly atmosphere. Dentists today must develop the ability to be flexible, intelligent and cooperative with their teams. These skills will move your practice forward in a cycle of continued growth, both emotionally and financially.

Take a moment to complete the following exercise to determine if your practice is ready to set the stage for a team environment.

Is your office suited for a Team environment?

(1) Circle or highlight the appropriate corresponding number, ranking each of the following characteristics of connected teams on a scale of 1 - 5. If any of these are nonexistent in your practice, then indicate it by marking "0," if you fully implement the characteristic then mark a "5."

(2) Take this survey a second time as a tool to indicate those characteristics that you *would like to implement* in your practice. Indicate these using a different color pen or highlighter.

Characteristic	Low					High

We have a shared vision that everyone knows, agrees on, and is committed to accomplishing.　　0　　1　　2　　3　　4　　5

We maintain a climate of trust and openness. Members feel involved and are willing to take risks.　　0　　1　　2　　3　　4　　5

We have open, honest communication. Members feel free to express their thoughts, feelings, and ideas. Each person listens and others feel free to put forth ideas without fear of embarrassment. Conflicts are viewed as natural and dealt with in an appropriate way.　　0　　1　　2　　3　　4　　5

A sense of belonging to the team. High-commitment and pride in the team's accomplishments exists.　　0　　1　　2　　3　　4　　5

Diversity is valued as an asset. People are viewed as unique and valuable resources. Flexibility and sensitivity to others is practiced.　　0　　1　　2　　3　　4　　5

Creativity and risk-taking are encouraged by the team leaders. Mistakes are viewed as a part of learning. Constant improvement can only take place if people are encouraged to try new ways.　　0　　1　　2　　3　　4　　5

Ability to self-correct. The team periodically looks at what may be interfering with its performance and develops solutions rather than letting problems worsen.　　0　　1　　2　　3　　4　　5

Members are interdependent.
They recognize that they need each other's knowledge,
skill, and resources to produce something they
could not do alone.   0   1   2   3   4   5

Consensus decision – making. Teams are making high
quality decisions and have the acceptance and support of the entire
team to carry them out.   0   1   2   3   4   5

Participative leadership. The leader of the group does not
dominate the group; instead, everyone
is viewed as a resource.   0   1   2   3   4   5

How does my team environment rank?

A score of: 0 – 20 indicates that team is not present in your practice.
Autocratic leadership seems to dominate.

21 – 30 indicates team presence, and there is room for
improvement. Isolate those areas ranking below
3 and mastermind ways to implement them in
your office at a level 5.
*Shift from autocratic to democratic leadership
is possible. Need guidance and coaching to
implement.*

31 – 40 indicates average to above average teams that
function well together. Several areas to improve
upon. Raise your standards and continue
implementation.
*Yes, your office is suited for a team environment.
Guidance and coaching in critical areas is needed.*

41 – 50 indicates team ownership and full accountability.
Peak performance level. Continue to monitor on
a routine basis.
*You have formed a strong and lasting team.
Coaching is indicated to continue successful
progress.*

Linda L. Miles, CSP, CMC
CEO, Miles & Associates

Linda has spent nearly two decades delivering her messages, building teams, and motivating practices across three continents. She has written four books, over 300 magazine and journal articles on practice management, and has produced numerous audio and video practice development programs.

From 1982 to 1987, Linda Miles & Associates grew by a phenomenal 544% and was named by Inc. magazine as one of the 500 fastest-growing, privately held companies in the United States. Miles & Associates is based in Virginia Beach, Virginia with associates located in Michigan, Hawaii, Florida, and New Jersey.

Linda's remarkable popularity and success is founded on the success of those who hear her and take her message to heart. You can contact Linda and her team of consultants by: Phone: (800) 922-0866, Fax: (757) 498-0290, or E-mail: LLMILES@ix.netcom.com

Words of Wisdom

During our monthly team meetings we review all production, collection and expense numbers, so each team member knows the financial status of the office and how that impacts their quarterly bonus. Each team member must know the financial health of the practice on a day to day basis.

DR. RANDY BOURJAILY
Novi, MI

We, as a group, created a bonus system that involved time-off with pay when the goal is achieved. Interestingly, this has been just as meaningful to the group as financial bonuses.

DR. PAUL KUHLMAN
Corunna, MI

We concentrate on things that go right! After a long stressful day, I find each team member and bring up a patient or situation they handled well. Asking them a question that focuses on what they did correctly gets them feeling good about themselves... and they float home remembering the one positive situation instead of the rest of the tough day.

DR. NEIL HOSS
Tolland, CT

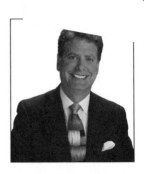

Chapter Two

'Polishing' your Relationships: Utilizing *The Platinum Rule* to Create Team Relationships

Nate Booth, D.D.S., M.S.

This is what it's all about: If you can't have fun at it, there's no sense hanging around. — JOE MONTANA

McGyver has just rescued the ambassador's daughter from the Colombian drug lords who were holding her captive. They have escaped to a small hut in the insect-infested jungle. The "bad guys" are closing in from all directions. The only "tools" McGyver has are his trusty Swiss Army Knife and a pack of chewing gum. Even though the situation looks worse than hopeless, McGyver always wins in the end. Why? Because McGyver understands the power of principles. He understands the principles of physics, chemistry, and mechanics. This understanding gives McGyver tremendous flexibility and power. He can be in any situation and use the resources around him to achieve his outcomes in life.

At the hut with McGyver and the ambassador's daughter we see this power in action. He notices the rear-view mirror on an old Jeep in the yard outside the hut. Taking the mirror, he creates a device that collects sunlight, concentrates it, and projects a ray of energy onto the bad guy's Mercedes, blowing it up just in the nick of time. Then he builds a transmitter using his Swiss Army Knife, chewing gum, and an ordinary radio. He calls his friends in Bagota and is rescued by helicopter just before the next wave of bad guys appears!

If you've ever watched McGyver, you know that I'm only slightly exaggerating. The point of this story is that McGyver utilizes the power of principles. Like McGyver, when you use the appropriate principles, you have the ability to be successful in a wide range of situations. The principles allow you to create the appropriate answer to almost every life question.

This chapter is about helping you understand and use one of the most vital principles I know — the principle of **The Platinum Rule.** We're all familiar with The Golden Rule, "Treat others the way you would like to be treated." The Golden Rule is certainly a powerful principle but it has one shortcoming: *everyone wants to be treated differently.* What may be excellent treatment to you, may or may not be excellent treatment to the staff and patients in your dental office. That's when The Platinum Rule comes into play. The Platinum Rule is, "Treat others in the unique way they want to be treated." When you apply The Platinum Rule to your dental office relationships, you will create a staff that will make your practice a masterpiece in action!

The definition of The Platinum Rule, "Treat others in the unique way they want to be treated," begs two questions:

What is it that people really want in life?

How can I discover what they really want in life?

Let's begin to answer these questions by playing a quick game. On a sheet of paper, write anything you want in your life. Now circle all your answers that are emotions such as love, security, or freedom. The answers you didn't circle are probably things or experiences such as money, a car, a home, a job, or a specific relationship. Next, answer this question about all the items you didn't circle. "If I had (the item you circled), it would give me (an emotion)." As an example, "If I had the home, it would give me happiness." Or "If I had $1,000,000, it would give me security." Or "If I had the relationship, it would give me love."

It always comes down to the feelings in the end. People don't want money. They want the feelings they think the money will give them. In fact, winning a million dollars in a lottery has screwed up many people's lives. The money not only didn't give the people the positive feelings they thought it would, it actually gave them pain in the long-term.

Question: What are the two best days of boat ownership? Many former boat owners would answer, "The day I bought it, and the day I sold it!" People don't want boats. They buy a boat thinking it will give them excitement or freedom. After the purchase, they discover it doesn't lead to the feelings they desired, and it's a pain in the rear to maintain. Then they sell it as soon as possible.

Unfortunately, cigarette manufacturers know that when it comes right down to it, people really want emotions. Take a close look at their advertisements some time. They never sell their product. They know that in reality their product has four main attributes: it's highly addictive; it's expensive; it stinks; and it kills people! Trying to push those four product features would be a "tough sale."

So, cigarette manufacturers don't sell cigarettes. They sell the emotions they know people want in their lives. They link one or more of these feelings to their brand of cigarette. Marlboro has done the most effective job of doing this and, as a result, is the most popular brand in the United States. What emotions do the makers of Marlboro say you will receive from using their product? Think about the scenes in their ads before you answer. A typical ad has a ruggedly handsome cowboy comfortably sitting by a campfire smoking a cigarette. It's only him, his horse, the beautiful natural surroundings, and his cigarette. The only other image in the picture is a big pack of Marlboro's down in the corner. The emotions Marlboro wants you to connect to their product are freedom, individualism, and contentment – three emotions highly valued by many people in our society.

Think about it for a second. How much sense does it really make to believe that becoming addicted to cigarettes will give you more freedom? Zero, zippo, none! But people don't do things for logical reasons. They do things for emotional reasons and sometimes justify their actions with logic. If people did things for logical reasons, men would be the ones riding sidesaddle! People do things for emotional reasons. People want emotions.

Now let's apply this information to life. Below are five emotions you may desire in your life. I could have listed hundreds, but I kept the list short to simplify the exercise. From this list, pick the one emotion that is most important — the one feeling you desire most in your life. If you have difficulty deciding between two emotions, ask yourself this question, "If I could only have one of these two emotions, which one would I choose?"

- Love
- Security
- Adventure
- Success
- Freedom

Continue to rank each of the four remaining emotions from most important to least important. Do this until you have the five emotions in order. The emotion you selected first is the one you value more than the others — your highest life value.

As you might imagine, not everyone would order the emotions the way you did, because people value emotions differently. Understanding these differences allows you to apply The Platinum Rule — to give people what they really want, in a way that they want it.

Let me share a personal example of Values in action. At one time, I was a very successful dentist. I had a huge dental practice and was making tons of money. But I absolutely hated being tied down to the "drilling, filling, and billing" of dentistry. So, I sold my practice and got out of the profession. Now, as a speaker and author, I choose the projects I want to work on and travel the world sharing ideas I believe in. For recreation, I frequently go scuba diving or do some other outdoor activity such as hiking, tennis, or golf. I've just shared a small slice of my life with you. I bet you now have a very good idea which of the five emotions I value most, and least, in life.

Freedom is at the top of my list. When I have freedom, I have the space to love others, be successful, and have adventure in my life. I'm attracted to jobs that give me freedom, sports that provide freedom, and other people who value freedom. My wife, Dawn, also puts freedom at the top of her list. Many times during the year I'll leave town for more than a week. Does Dawn cuddle up to me as I'm walking out the door and whisper gently in my ear, "I really wish you didn't have to go." Heck no! She says, "See ya! Don't call home 'cause I probably won't be here!" Our relationship works well because we have a #1 Value in common.

What emotion of the five do you think would be lowest on my list? If you guessed security, you're absolutely correct. Security doesn't appeal to me at all. When things get too secure in my life, I consciously and unconsciously shake things up!

Here's an example of the danger of not knowing someone's Values. Occasionally, I'll talk to a financial planner who is trying to sell an investment plan. What emotion do you think he tries to sell me nine times out of ten? Security! It's truly amazing and amusing to see the sales process unfold. In the beginning of the sales call, the planner will ask me, "At what age do you want to retire?" I answer, "Retire from what? I never want to retire. I'm having too much fun in my life to retire!"

You should see the look on his face. He doesn't know what to do now. It completely screws up his sales presentation because he can't pull out his handy-dandy little chart that shows how much money I need to put away each year to comfortably retire at age 65. Then he will say something that sounds to me like, "Well, don't you want to build a nest egg so you can retire in Yuma, Arizona, in a old person depository and play shuffleboard every afternoon and bingo on Wednesday evenings?" What do I think of that vision of the future? It makes me sick. I want to keep "working" until I drop and eventually have a fantastic place in the mountains where my family and I can ski, hike, bike, and enjoy all the freedom the world has to offer! If the financial planner would sell me freedom, I would be all ears.

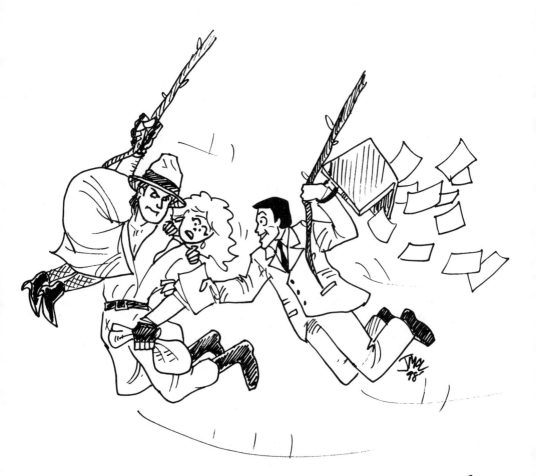

You <u>MUST</u> RELATE TO SOMEONE'S VALUES

Discovering a Person's Values

To discover a person's Values, follow this simple, yet profound, advice, "Ask and you shall receive." You will be amazed at what people will tell you if you establish even a moderate level of rapport and trust. To be an effective Values detective, follow these two steps:

Ask the Values Questions, "What's most important to you in (the Values Area you want to explore)?" The exact question you ask will be determined by your relationship with the person and the areas you want to explore. If you want to discover a patient's most important value in a relationship with your practice ask, "What's most important to you in a relationship with our dental practice?" With a co-worker, "What's most important to you in a relationship with a teammate?"

If you want to discover a second Value for a particular Values Area, ask, "What else is important to you in (the Values Area you want to explore)?" As an example, "What else is important to you in a relationship with a teammate?"

Have you ever played a game with someone and each of you had a different set of rules for the game? What happened when you played the game for a period of time? There was some conflict, right? Both of you became upset because the other person didn't know the rules of the game. To keep the game going, you had to reach an agreement on the rules in question.

The same thing happens in real life, every day, in your practice. Even if you have a common set of Values, each of you has a personal set of rules concerning relationships and how they "should" work. Because people are different, the two sets of rules are probably different. Unless you get clear on the rules, you too will have conflict.

The word we use for rules is "Sparks." Sparks are the things that have to happen for people to experience their Values. Each person's unique set of Sparks determines how he wants to play the relationship "game" with you.

By giving people what they really want in life is more than just avoiding conflict. It's proactively discovering what people want (their Values) and how they want it (their Sparks, or rules). Now you can give them what they want in the way they want it on a consistent basis.

Here's an example of Values and Sparks in action. Love is a Value that is very high on most people's Values lists. It is for my wife, Dawn, and me. If you've ever been in love, you know that different people have different Sparks for what has to happen for each other to feel love. In our relationship, I could never tell Dawn I love her, and it wouldn't bother her one bit! It's not one of her Sparks for love. She feels love when we go places and do things together — when we share experiences. If you're shaking your head in disapproval right now, it just means that you have different Sparks for love than Dawn. If you're agreeing with me, it means that you have the same Rule for love as Dawn. I want my wife to feel loved. So, what do I do on a regular basis? I plan trips where we go places and do things together.

The purpose of this chapter is not to help you examine your personal Values and Sparks, (although I hope I've stimulated your interest). The point of this chapter is to help you understand the principles of Values and Sparks, the power of The Platinum Rule, and how to discover other people's Values and Sparks.

To get the most out of this chapter, it is vital that you begin putting The Platinum Rule into action as soon as possible. That's why I've placed exercises for action at the end of the chapter. I strongly recommend that you use this section as the focal point for one or more of your staff meetings.

Discovering a Person's Sparks

After you have learned a person's first Value with the Values Question, you can discover his Spark for that Value. Ask the Sparks Question: "What has to happen in order for you to feel (the Value you just discovered)?" In Dawn's case it would be, "What has to happen in order for you to feel loved." Her first rule is "When we go places."

There may be multiple Sparks for each Value. To discover these additional Sparks, ask the question, "What else has to happen in order for you to feel (the Value you just discovered)?"

The question can be worded differently depending on the situation. For Dawn, her second rule was "to share experiences." It's not enough that we happen to be in the same place at the same time. She needs to feel that we are "sharing experiences."

There are many ways to word Values and Sparks Questions. The exact wording is not as important as making The Platinum Rule a way of life. Living a life based on discovering what people want and how they want it, then giving it to them when it's in their best long-term interest will bring you the emotions you desire and deserve.

Discovering Values and Sparks for Team Members

As a leader, it's vital that you create a compelling common goal that inspires people. It is equally vital that you use The Platinum Rule to understand the diverse group of people in your office, align them according to their unique and valuable roles, and understand their different reasons for working with you. The best definition of a team I've ever seen is, "A team is a diverse group of people, each with a unique and valuable role, gathered together for a common goal, for different reasons."

With your dental office associates, you will want to explore three Values Areas:

1. The Job/Occupation Values Area
2. The Relationship with Teammates Area
3. The Life Values Area

Explore each of these by first asking, "What's most important to you in a job/occupation?" For example, with your hygienist, you might ask "What is most important to you in being a hygienist?" With a supplier "What's most important to you in being a dental supply representative?" With your referral network "What is most important to you about being a (type of specialist)?" Discover his/her #1 Value for this area.

After discovering the Value, ask, "What has to happen in order for you to feel (#1 Value)?" In the example with a hygienist, let's say her #1 for being a hygienist is "respected as a professional," ask "What has to happen in order for you to feel you are respected as a professional?"

Continue to ask the Values and Sparks pertaining to job/occupation questions until you have discovered two or three primary Values. You can then move into areas of team relationships and life values.

Let me illustrate this process by sharing a composite of conversations I have had with work associates through the years. I have used this as an invaluable and successful interviewing technique for many years.

Nate   "Mary, I really like to get to know the people I work within the dental office because everyone has different wants and needs. Would you mind answering a few questions?"

Mary   "Sounds good to me."

Nate   "What's most important to you in a job?"

Mary   "Oh, I don't know. Making lots of money, I guess." (A vague Spark answer.)

Nate   "If you made lots of money, what would that mean to you?" (I'm elevating her Spark to a Value.)

Mary   "That would mean I'm successful." (A Value of hers. It may or may not be her highest Value.)

Nate   "How much money would you have to make this year to feel like you're successful?" (I'm getting more specific on her Spark for success.)

Mary   "$30,000."

Nate   "Let's see. You make $25,000 now. I've got some ideas of skills you can learn that could lead to an improved income. When we have some more time, we can review a few of them."

Mary   "Great!" (People get excited when they feel understood and supported.)

Nate   "What else has to happen for you to feel success?" (I'm after her second Spark for success.)

Mary   "Hmmmm, being recognized for the good work I do." (Her second Spark for success.)

Nate   "There's a lot of ways to be recognized. Which ways are important to you?" (I'm getting very clear on this Spark.)

Mary   "It doesn't have to be anything formal. Although that's OK. I just like to be told every once in a while that I'm doing a good job."

Moving onto her second Value for Job/Occupation, I ask:

Nate   "In addition to success, what else is important to you in a job?"

Mary   "I want a job that challenges me." (Challenge is her second Value)

Nate   "Of the two things you've mentioned so far — success and challenge — which one is most important to you?" (I want to discover her #1 Value.)

Mary   "That's a good question."

Nate   "What's a good answer?"

Mary   "Probably challenge."

Nate   "How does a job have to be arranged for it to be challenging?" (Another way of asking for a Spark.)

Mary   "I need to be constantly learning." (Her first Spark for challenge.)

Nate   "What are a few things you would like to learn now that would help you the most?" (I want to discover how I can help her right now. When I do that, I'll have an eager and hard-working dental associate.)

Mary   "Whoa, you'd do that for me?"

Nate   "Within reason, whenever and wherever I can."

Mary   "I need to learn the new accounting program we use here in the office."

Nate   "That's a good first choice. I'll get you enrolled in the next full day training class. After you've completed the class, we'll talk about the next step."

Mary   "I really appreciate your time. I've never worked for someone who took the time to find out what I was thinking before. It feels nice to be heard."

Nate   "This is the type of open communication you can always count on from me."

Now let's move into the second Values Area — relationship with teammates.

Nate   "I'm curious. What's most important to you in a relationship with a teammate?"

Mary   She answers very quickly and with a fair amount of intensity "Respect." (Her first Value for this Value Area.)

Nate "It didn't take you long to answer. Did you ever work in a dental office where you didn't feel respected?" (I knew from the way she answered my last question that in a previous position, she probably felt disrespected.)

Mary "You bet. I quit my last job because I wasn't given any respect."

Nate "You sound like Rodney Dangerfield. Do you think the problem was with you or them?"

Mary "What do you mean by that?"

Nate "Sometimes people have such unrealistic expectations of how other people should act that they're never satisfied no matter what situation they're in."

Mary "Whooooa, I never thought of it like that. Maybe I have been a little overboard with my expectations."

Nate "That's just something to think about. In the mean time, what can I do to let you know you're respected?" (Another form of Sparks Question. Remember that this whole process is more than just asking a series of questions; it's a way of thinking.)

Mary "When you give me an assignment, don't be constantly looking over my shoulder." (She states her Spark in the negative.)

Nate "You've told me what you don't want me to do. Tell me what you do want me to do."

Mary "When you give me an assignment, let me run with it."

Nate "Be a little more specific. What does 'let me run with it' mean?"

Mary "It means that you never bother me about it or ask me how I'm doing." (It looks like some of her unrealistic expectations are coming out again. Just because somebody says that she wants to be treated in a certain way doesn't mean that you must do it. As in this case, maybe you have to educate the person a little or compromise.)

Nate "Mary, I appreciate your independence. We need independent thinkers around here; however, I'm responsible for the results of this office. I need to know what's going on so I can help you if I can and coordinate the efforts of the other people in the office with what you're doing. How can we arrange it so I get the information I need, and you feel respected?"

Mary "Yeah, I see what you mean. How about if I give you a written report of how I'm doing every Friday?"

Nate "That sounds fine. I'll be expecting it each Friday. In addition, how about if I just stick my head in every week or so to see how

you're doing? I'm not trying to be Big Brother or anything;
I just want to make sure we're all moving in roughly the same
direction. And if you ever want to try something that's in a
completely different direction, let me know, and I'll see what
I can do. Of course, my door is always open to you if you have
any questions or need some resources."

Mary "That sounds fair." (We've negotiated the rules of the game.)

After discovering several other Values and Sparks for relationships
with teammates, I then move on to discover those for the Life Area.
You may have noticed that we always start with the less personal Job/
Occupation Values Area and move progressively through the
Relationship with Teammates Values Area to the more personal Life
Values Area. By so structuring your conversation, you invite the other
person to "open up."

Can you see the benefit in discovering what people want (Values)
and how they want it (Sparks)? This is much more than a series of
questions. It is a shift in your mindset, which will enable you to be
much more precise in your ability to form deep relationships that last. It
will also help you to communicate with your team because you will
"see where they're coming from." You will understand their unique set
of desires that are probably different from your own. Understanding the
diversity of people's desires will stimulate creativity in your team
because members will feel free to express their ideas and explore
different ways of accomplishing their daily tasks.

You will be able to more easily solve upsets when they occur because
you will have a common Values and Sparks language to discuss the
upset. The ability to consistently and precisely give people what they
want, in the way they want it, will absolutely minimize staff turnover and
create a top performance team, ready to serve your patients.

Nate Booth, D.D.S., M.S.

Nate Booth, D.D.S., M.S., is the top Corporate Trainer for the Anthony Robbins Companies. He is the author of <u>The Platinum Touch: How to Give People what They Uniquely Desire</u> and <u>Thriving on Change: The Art of Using Change to Your Advantage.</u> He is the co-creator of the dental office study program, <u>Elegant Influence: The Art of Influencing Patients to Say "Yes!"</u> Please call (800) 917-0008 or E-mail: <u>nbooth@natebooth.com</u> for more information.

Words of Wisdom 🦷

We… ask for help and volunteer to help each other in our morning huddle.

DR. B.B. BUSKIRK
Gig Harbor, WA

Continually recognize superior performance and acknowledge commitment beyond the call of duty. Reinforcing those activities that allow the team to reach higher standards.

DR. JEFF PRILUCK AND DR. AL NORDONE
Dunwoody, GA

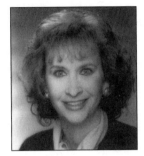

Chapter Three

'Filling' Openings in Your Team Roster: Tips on Hiring, Training Top Performers, And Dismissing Non-Team Players

Carol Hacker

"Among the chief worries of today's business executives is the large number of unemployed still on the payrolls." ANONYMOUS

The hiring process is the most critical step in forming your peak performance team. The right hiring decision creates the difference between heaven and heartache. Here are some tips for choosing the right candidate for your office.

Tips on Hiring

Make a list of qualities you are looking for in each position of the practice. Continually seek new employees. In growing organizations, there is always room for outstanding people to contribute to your team. Hire only ACE employees: positive Attitude, great Communication skills, and Enthusiasm.

Conduct pre-screening interviews by telephone.

Gather information rather than give information — the number one mistake hiring managers' make is talking too much during the interview.

Ask permission to take notes during the interview.

Check a minimum of three work-related references. Personal references are worthless.

Have highly potential candidates work for 1– 3 days as part of a working interview.

Have the staff take highly potential candidates out for lunch (preferably at a restaurant with wait staff) to observe their interaction with others, and to get to know them on a personal level.

Use the first two weeks as a trial period, whereby either the candidate or the practice can terminate the relationship with no hard feelings. Let the candidate also know that you will continue to interview during this time.

Training Top Performers

Once you've made your selection, training is critical. It has been my experience that most practices throw new employees into the "deep-end." This becomes especially true when the candidate has a comprehensive background and experience. Regardless of previous experience, new employees need to become familiar with your office policies, and culture. Here are some quick training tips to integrate new staff into your practice.

Ask new employees to review the Vision Statement, Agreements, Policies, and Procedures of the practice. There should be a written acknowledgment of agreement to support and adhere to these policies filed in their personnel folder.

Define your Top Three Priorities for each position.

Prepare clearly defined job description.

Designate a mentor to guide new staff as they become integrated into the practice.

Have clearly defined and understood tasks with time table for competency in place during the learning cycle.

Review progress frequently.

Encourage new staff to ask questions!

At the end of 90 days have the entire staff conduct a review of performance and competency. Identify areas that need extra attention for the next 90 days.

Throughout the training process, praise and encourage new staff. This creates a relaxed environment that is conducive to learning.

Utilize Standard Operating Procedures Manual as a central place to record the "correct" way to perform tasks. Update this as procedures change, to simplify training tasks (especially for large group, or multi-location practices.)

Dismissing Non-Team Players

We've all experienced the anguish of dismissing an employee. I would like to share a new philosophy with you. In highly developed Top Performance Teams, there are often agreements in place similar to this:

1. No staff member shall leave the practice, without first securing a replacement of equal or greater ability.

2. No employee shall be dismissed from the practice without assisting in locating another position in a suitable office. Can you imagine the impact these two agreements would have on your team's morale and sense of security?

Regardless of whether you adopt these agreements, there may come a point in time when it is evident that someone does not belong on your team. Here are some tips for making the transition easier.

Before you terminate — consider the degree of the offense, look at the employees' length of services, and past dedication to the team.

Decide whether or not the office rules and policies have been consistently applied.

Avoid dismissals due to emotional upset by applying the communication technology you have learned in this book.

When someone is not acting in a way that supports the vision and agreements of your practice, have a frank discussion with them. Outline specific performance criteria, and give them 30 days notice to improve performance.

Refer to your office SOP (standard operating procedure) regarding disciplinary action and termination. Be consistent.

Document all conversations relating to job performance and disciplinary action in personnel records.

Recognize the difference between an employee who needs "emotional first aid" and one who *should* be fired.

Remember, when you dismiss someone, you also dismiss his/her family. Whenever possible, assist in finding another position.

Write letters of recommendation that speak to the performance of the individual, and whether you would rehire this person based on your experience as an employer.

At time of termination, have the employee turn in all keys, uniforms, and related office property. Deliver final paycheck and letter of recommendation (if appropriate) once all property has been returned.

Carol Hacker

Carol is an educator, speaker and the founder of Carol A. Hacker & Associates, one of the country's foremost skill-building enterprises on human resource management. For more than two decades she's been a significant voice in front-line and corporate human resource management to Fortune 500 companies as well as small businesses. She's a graduate of the University of Wisconsin, where she earned her B.S. and M.S. with honors.

Carol is the author of the highly acclaimed books, <u>Hiring Top Performers — 350 Great Interview Questions For People Who Need People</u> (1994), <u>The Costs of Bad Hiring Decisions & How to Avoid Them</u> (St. Lucie Press 1996; 2nd edition 1998), <u>The High Cost of Low Morale… and what to do about it.</u> (St. Lucie Press 1997), and dozens of published articles.

She's a member of the National Speakers Association, Georgia Speakers Association, and speaks for professional and trade associations, as well as for private corporations and government agencies. Her motivational presentations are practical, positive, and entertaining. Her interactive workshops have helped thousands of managers become better leaders.

Carol is available to speak at companies, association meetings, or to consult with organizations on the topics of selecting and keeping winning employees. For more information please call (770) 410-0517, Fax (770) 667-9801, or E-mail: <u>GaonMind@aol.com</u>

Words of Wisdom 🦷

We treat each member equally, and we support each other when we have family problems-like sick kids, parents, etc.

DR. BORRIS BRIDGET
Las Cruces, NM

It's the attitude of the willingness to "go the extra mile" for each other that is the crux of the success of the team. There is nothing each one of us won't do for another. Also, having a sense of humor and light heartedness helps.

DR. HERBERT K. LAND
Raleigh, NC

We all are sensitive to each other's feelings. If one person needs help, we all pitch in. We work together to provide a good working atmosphere, not only for ourselves, but our patients as well.

ROSSETTI DENTAL
New Albany, MS

Consistency and diligence by the head coach work to create certainty and safety in developing teams. They need to know that they can depend on certain qualities, abilities, and behavior from their coach (boss) 100% of the time.

DR. MICHAEL R. EGAN
Hartford, CT

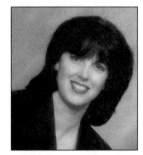

Chapter Four

'Flossing' over Conflict?
Effective Strategies for Dealing with Conflict

Brenda Kaesler, RDH

"The Constitution only guarantees the American people the right to pursue happiness. You have to catch it yourself." — BENJAMIN FRANKLIN

It was her first day as a new dental assistant in our practice. Not having been part of the interview or selection process, I hadn't been introduced to her until right before I had to seat my first patient. "Jeni," as we'll call her, seemed all right — after all, how could I really judge her in that one brief introduction? As I was cleaning my patient's teeth, Jeni entered my operatory, mounting a full mouth series I had taken the day before. She quickly proclaimed, "When you take a full mouth series, if you get a cone cut, you *must* retake the x-ray." Jeni had been on my team for less than 30 minutes and the turf war that turned out to last close to a year had begun!

I wish I could tell you that I confronted the situation in a calm, timely, empowering, responsible (or at least semi-adult) sort of way. Nope! I went into a full out, calculated, around the flanks assault that should have cost me my job, and did cost me, our team and the dentist months of fulfillment. How dare she come into our practice, much less into my operatory, and correct me in front of my patient! Obviously, she doesn't have our values, play by our rules, or actually belong on our team. My life became about removing her from "our" turf! Now, many years later, I can look back and understand that I owe quite a bit to Jeni — not to mention the doctor who tolerated me during this time of what I like to call "growth." Going through that conflict helped me understand more about group dynamics, such as conflict is internally, not externally, generated. Jeni helped me understand that it isn't even necessary to like the people on your team as long as you stay focused on an outcome that is bigger than yourself. In addition, the experience with Jeni demonstrated the incredible importance of having a leader who is committed to the growth of the individuals and the organization.

Historically, we have viewed conflict and confrontation as something to be avoided at all cost. That's because most of us don't have enough references of conflict as exciting, energizing, and beneficial. We haven't yet learned to embrace conflict as an opportunity to learn about other people or as a way to deepen our relationships. We see conflict as painful and demoralizing, and truthfully, most of the time it turns out that way. It's no wonder we run from conflict as fast as we can! In fact, when I ask people to list their number one most painful emotional state, something they will do almost anything to avoid, conflict and confrontation heads the list the majority of the time. Since we haven't been given the training to recognize conflict in its early cycle or the tools to turn it into a powerful force for good, most of our conflicts deteriorate into painful experiences, reinforcing our inability to address situations.

Conflict is an inevitable part of human interaction, whether it is inspired by diverse personalities, style, rules, or expectations, and whether it surfaces as outright war or played out in a more covert, undermining scenario. Ultimately, early diagnosis and implementation of a straightforward action plan can channel the negative conflict into a powerful tool for growth and positive change.

Conflict Origination

Most upsets come from one of two domains, unfulfilled expectations or frustrated intentions. An *expectation* is an outcome that you anticipate from others, and an *intention* is an outcome you anticipate from yourself. During dental school a dentist has a dream of what life after school will be like. The usual scenarios highlight starting a private practice, buying an existing practice, or becoming a temporary associate in someone else's practice. His or her dreams are heavy with intended outcomes and expectations. Let's use these examples:

I will attract only the patients who want the best dentistry.
(intended outcome)

When I tell the patients what's best, they will automatically schedule and pay for the treatment. (expectation)

My staff will be committed, highly motivated individuals who never argue, will work for minimum wage, and never complain about staying late. (expectation)

Even if your diagnostic skills are rusty, you can find at least three areas for big-time conflict, and we haven't even gotten out of school yet! These intentions and expectations are most likely destined to remain unfulfilled and frustrated somewhere during the odyssey of practicing dentistry.

The specific expectations and intentions, however, are irrelevant. The point is that there will be breakdowns in the process of accomplishing any outcome. When our intentions are not met, or our expectations are unfulfilled, most of us allow ourselves to become frustrated. Maybe just a little frustrated at first, but if we aren't skilled in mastering our own internal conversations, an internal conflict ignites. We usually don't resolve this type of conflict in a positive way. Perhaps we begin by lashing out, either consciously or unconsciously, at those people who are actually there to support us. For instance, I was recently in the office of a doctor we will call "Tim" who complained of feeling pressured and irritable and admitted that he had been lashing out at his staff. He thought it was because his numbers were down; but, in fact, they were up. During the quest to pinpoint the specific unfulfilled expectation or frustrated intention, we uncovered that he felt "out of control" with his operative patients. To make a short story shorter — three months earlier, he decided to change his new patient examination protocol and see all new patients in the hygiene department. This one change, and the way it was handled, created huge amounts of uncertainty for Tim (frustrated intention.) He had begun lashing out at his staff, and, even worse, at his patients. This compounded the negative feelings because the patient's expectations of being treated nicely became unfulfilled, and so goes the cycle. Stop now and think of any conflict you are currently experiencing, or have recently experienced. Determine if the *root* of the conflict was an unfulfilled expectation or a frustrated intention, as you read on, determine the *type* of conflict. (Remember an expectation is an outcome that you anticipate from others, and an intention is an outcome you anticipate from yourself.)

Types of Conflict

There are three basic types of conflicts:

1. *Interpersonal* — which involves a conflict with another person. This may be because of differences in personality, in opinion, rules, knowledge, or values. Whatever its source, the conflict resolution will most likely focus on resolving personal issues with the other party. It is extremely important to resolve personal differences when the parties involved in the conflict interact in a close working relationship! My conflict with Jeni was mostly interpersonal.

2. *Organizational* — this type of conflict involves a conflict with policies, procedures, internal politics, or organizational structure. These conflicts could relate to: starting on time, getting out for lunch routinely, running late at the end of the day, running out of certain supplies, unproductive schedules, etc. Tim's conflict was organizational because it related to procedure and protocol.

3. *Environmental* — this conflict involves sources outside the organization. These sources could include insurance companies, capitation plans, the "low dental IQ syndrome," shortage of hygienists, shortage of excellent chairside assistants, restrictive laws, etc.

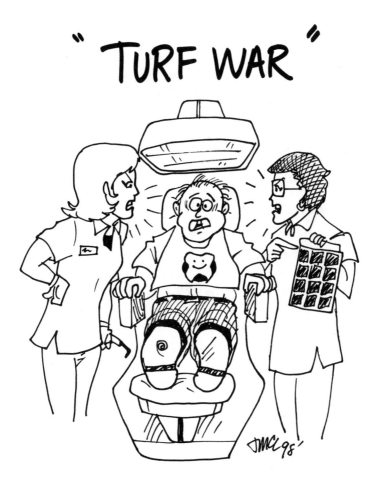

"TURF WAR"

RESOLVE CONFLICTS IN EARLY STAGES!

Diagnosis is the first step in handling conflict quickly and painlessly. Granted, we don't seem to have trouble determining conflict when it is a raging and bloody war! It is the subtle, early warning signs that go undetected and unconfronted. It's like the hygienist scaling her knuckles off in 5mm pockets, charging for a prophy, and preaching to the patient that they should floss their teeth more often! The disease is seen, possibly not recognized for what it is (undiagnosed), and certainly not confronted. The early signs and symptoms of conflict can be confusing and somewhat invisible, just like periodontal disease. And, just as damaging! Conflict, if left untreated, will result in low energy, loss of productivity, loss of patience, loss of patients, and the loss of good team members.

Let's dissect my conflict with Jeni. Before Jeni became part of our organization, we had a great team of people working together to accomplish common goals; we had synergy going for us. You could say that we made it all the way through the stages of team building and we were peak performers. Then, one of our dental assistants moved. My expectation of a new dental assistant was that she would automatically step into the shoes of our peak performer in all aspects including relationship and technical skills, compassion, and passion, and drive for what we were accomplishing as a team. Never once did I think that we would literally have to start over, to rebuild our team, to stop and get to know the idiosyncrasies of another human being, or allow her time to get to know ours. Looking back, it seems quite obvious; but, when we are in the game, it's difficult to step back, take a look, and practice the basics! So, some thirty minutes into our game, Jeni became my enemy. All because my unreasonable expectations were not fulfilled.

The Rules

It's simple to see the breakdown and what the simple treatment should have been. As Nate said earlier, we all have conditions or "rules" that we attach to relationships and events in our lives. These rules are based on previous life experiences, or social conditioning.

Looking back at my experience with Jeni, I can see what really happened. Jeni was new and probably a little bit nervous. She had excellent qualifications as a technical assistant, and part of the strength she could bring to our practice was the regimentation she was accustomed to as an Army dental assistant. At the time, we were lacking systematic clinical protocols, and she was the one to augment this area. Her extremely high personal standards of treatment quality spilled over into every aspect, including the absence of cone cuts on x-rays. While cone cuts were high on her list of rules, I, on the other hand, viewed them as a perfect way to educate the patients on the minimal amount of scatter radiation that exists in dental x-rays. I know, you really *shouldn't* get a cone cut on an x-ray; but, make it work for you if it happens. Get the picture? The lack of a cone cut was low on my list of rules! I was the first person on our team to break one of Jeni's most important rules. As a consequence, Jeni's brain immediately registered two immediate responses — the questions of evaluation that every single one of us asks with every event that occurs — "What does this mean?" (Substandard x-rays) and "What should I do?" (correct the behavior immediately so it doesn't happen again). That's what she did, which violated one of my highest rules… you <u>must never</u> criticize or correct anyone in front of patients. It wasn't the fact that she had corrected me because believe me, I was really used to corrections, and most of the time I was able to see them as performance-based, not personal. However, her breaking my rule sent me into orbit.

I now attempt to operate from the belief, shared with me by Anthony Robbins, *"All communication is either a loving response or a cry for help."* When a rule is violated, which type of communication do you think we demonstrate? If you choose a cry for help as the answer, you are catching onto the reason for conflict! When one of our rules is violated, we react with a cry for help, either lashing out, or withholding communication, but rarely with a loving response. And because we don't catch on quickly, the next step in the cycle of conflict results in justifying our upset and further distancing ourselves from reality.

Perhaps the most important concept in this chapter is: in order to deal effectively with challenges, team members need to understand the anatomy of upsets and be well-equipped and well-trained in communication. Initially, someone must intervene and direct conflict into an empowering interaction, otherwise, the situation could get ugly. When people don't deal with their upsets quickly, they will find someone who will take their side in the justification process. You know what I am saying here. This is the "grapevine," the "office gossip," the "sub-grouping," that takes place in most offices on a daily basis. Create strong agreements within your team to prevent this type of interoffice gossip.

Changing Your Interpretations

How do you change interpretations of events? By simply discovering the negative meaning you've attached to a situation and replacing them with positive, more powerful meanings. Of course, if you really are committed to drama and upset, feel free to keep your disempowering and probably inaccurate meanings. Stop now and think about a current conflict and its cause:

1. An event takes place, and you ask the question:
   a. "What does this mean?"
2. You attach certain meanings to the event, then you ask:
   b. "What should I do?"

Take that same conflict, and add some new questions:
1. Remember the event and ask:
   a. What does this mean?
2. You attach certain meanings to the event, then you ask:
   b. "Does this meaning empower me and others involved?"
3. If the answer is "no," then you ask:
   c. "What else could this mean that would empower me and others involved?"
4. Now you can ask:
   d. "What can I do that will meet my needs and the needs of others involved?"

So, how did it wind up with Jeni and me? After about nine months of battle cries and injuries, Doc finally had enough and scheduled a meeting to handle "the situation." Holding two boxes of Kleenex, he stated that we were staying until it got resolved. Ultimately, we agreed to disagree, learned about each other's intentions, and committed to working together. We both decided nothing was worth the trauma we put ourselves through, and nothing could bring back the nine months we had wasted being upset.

Strategies to Minimize Conflict

Create very clear and specific expectations of performance. This creates certainty for you and the staff member.

Set goals & challenges. People are fulfilled when they are growing and contributing. Providing an environment for these needs to be met will focus people on something bigger than their own personalities.

Act quickly when confronting disagreements. Allowing any source of upset to interfere with your outcomes drains your team energy.

Involve people in developing and implementing strategies that will move challenging situations past the breakdown that occurs.

Upgrade skills continuously. Provide pertinent, continuous training to give your staff the tools to be productive and contributing members of the team. Communication and relationship training is as important as clinical and training.

Recognize that pride drives performance more than money. Every team member needs to be acknowledged for his/her contributions to the organization. The absence of demonstrated gratitude results in the abundance of interpersonal conflict.

Establishing the Rules for Confrontation

Here is an effective team exercise for establishing ground rules for open honest communication. It is recommended that each person individually answer each statement true or false. Then, as a team, rate each one true or false. On any with less than a unanimous response, discuss the topic until consensus is reached.

T or F   1. A team member should feel free to say anything he/she has on his/her mind.

T or F   2. Unless requested, a team member should not give feedback.

T or F   3. A better tactic is to not participate in a discussion then to pursue an issue that could lead to confrontation.

T or F   4. Team unity is what matters more than anything else.

T or F   5. It's possible for team members to be *too nice.*

T or F   6. Being emotional or getting personal is not healthy under any circumstances.

T or F   7. If you work at it long enough you can always come to agreement.

T or F   8. Sometime conflict can actually feel exhilarating.

T or F   9. When trust is high conflict is low.

T or F   10. A healthy and fair approach is to let the doctor settle all disputes.

T or F   11. Conflict is a useless waste of time and energy.

T or F   12. A team should have rules for handling conflict.

T or F   13. You must have a good relationship with every member of the team.

T or F   14. If consensus is reached, every member of the team must abide by the decision.

Brenda Kaesler, RDH

Brenda's commitment to building productive, profitable, and fulfilling dental practices spans a career of over 20 years. As a practicing hygienist, she mastered the art of selling dentistry by building communication skills that influence patients to take responsibility for their own dental health. As a consultant with Fortune Practice Management®— Dallas, she has helped hundreds of practices implement these strategies and build teams that provide high quality care and bottom-line results. As a communications trainer and coach, she has assisted thousands of people in learning effective and empowering approaches to settling and working through conflict and confrontation.

A graduate of Tyler University School of Dental Hygiene, in Tyler, Texas, she has taken her dynamic repertoire of training programs across the United States and Canada speaking to dentists on topics ranging from Communication to Marketing, and the full range of practice management topics. She is the co-creator of the dental office case presentation program, Elegant Influence: The Art of Influencing Patients to say "Yes!" She resides with her husband and two children in San Diego, CA and can be reached at (760) 727-4509 or E-mail: FPMDALLAS@compuserve.com

Words of Wisdom 🦷

We have never been ones to buy into gimmicks or quick-fixes, therefore, we try to promote each other on a daily basis. We promote each other through supporting, encouraging, and developing each other as team members and also as persons. There are eight of us, but we feel as if we are one.

DR. DAVID A. DUNCAN
Amarillo, TX

[We have] the ability of all the staff to comfortably fill in or cover a position in the office that's vacant due to illness or other reasons.

DR. RICHARD S. WILSON
Richmond, VA

(For the past six years!) We have a personal trainer two days per week come to our office for free weights and step aerobics. The exercise is great and we have a lot of laughs. It's fun, healthy, and convenient. The office pays half of the fee per session.

DR. HARVEY KERSTIEN
Clearwater, FL

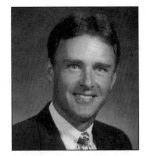

Chapter Five

Are there 'Open Margins' in your Team? Creating the Context of your Team

A. Paul Bass, III, D.D.S.

"The price of greatness is responsibility." — WINSTON S. CHURCHILL

If I could share one thing with you that would take your team to the next level of performance, it would be to recreate, or rethink, the structure of the team. Think of a glass of water. Every glass of water has two primary parts — the glass and its content, the water. Let's think of your practice as this glass of water. The water is representative of everything that you *do* within your practice. The truth is every healthcare provider — whether in dentistry, chiropractic, general medicine, opthalmology, or obstetrics — performs routine tasks daily. Thus, we all provide treatment, schedule appointments, collect fees, file insurance, reactivate patients, and so on. Regardless of the type of dental practice, you have the same content (water) as the dental practice down the street. We all *do* the same things.

The distinguishing factor then is the context of the team, your glass. If you take the same H_2O molecules and place them in a jelly jar, they assume a shape different from that of a champagne flute. The same is true for your practice — the context of your team determines your appearance to the outside world.

There are four components of your team's context — vision, agreements, communication, and relationships. These elements make up the *being* aspect of our practice, and define how we interact with one another and our patients. Without each of these elements in its proper place, you'll have a hole in your glass. And at that point, it really doesn't matter what you do; the results will never take form. Like pouring water through a colander, it's not what we *do* that makes a difference; it's how we *be*.

For the team, the real questions are: "How are we? Where do we currently stand on a scale from 1-10, (10 being Top Performance)?" Where do we need to be in order to have an outstanding team?

The first element in creating your context is the vision. What every team needs is a shared vision. This means that it is not just the doctor's vision. If it is, who is committed to supporting it? That's right, just the doctor. Every member of your team must be a part of creating a shared vision. As new people come on board, they must adopt this vision and take it on fully, or they are not aligned with your team. Your vision must also be an expanding vision. We are only effective when we are growing. Each year, review your vision statement and find ways to expand it to continue the cycle of growth.

In order to fulfill your vision, you must have supportive agreements. One thing to establish is that we can count on each other. What is it like to have a relationship with someone that you flat-out know you can count on? Think of someone in your life right now who is like that. Doesn't this give you the feeling of security, stability, peace, and contentment? If you want this type of relationship in your practice, you must design agreements that support the vision and design of your practice.

Think for a moment about the emotions and feelings you want to experience on a daily basis. This is the foundation of creating your vision, and as your vision expands, your agreements expand accordingly. The key to your team's moving to the next level is maintaining your agreements on a consistent basis.

Look at each agreement, evaluate at what level each is being met? If you do not have agreements in place that support your vision, you have a hole in your glass. How many holes does it take to lose your water? How many agreements have to be out of place in order to lose the integrity of your team?

One agreement I invite you to adopt is to support one another in keeping your agreements. There will be days when someone on your team just does not feel like keeping his or her agreements. If you intend to be outstanding, then you must support one another in keeping agreements. On a day when someone shows up with difficulty in keeping agreements, you must support her that day, remembering that tomorrow you may be the one needing support. Also, when you have a weed in your garden what do you do? Do you handle it when you first see it, or do you wait until it has overtaken the garden? It is up to each of us to keep the weeds out. You see the weed has its own agreement, to strangle the healthy vegetation and perpetuate its survival. It's not about right or wrong; it's simply a matter of function.

Establish agreements that keep the weeds out. One of those agreements is to take our concerns and upsets only to the person who can do something about them. I invite you also to establish an agreement to redirect others who share upsets that have nothing to do with you, otherwise known as gossip or sub-grouping. This type of communication in a practice is a weed, which we must eliminate to keep our garden healthy.

The third part of your context is communications. Communication must be open, honest, and supportive. The word "open" implies that anyone can talk to anyone honestly and constructively. But not all communication is of this nature. Sometimes it is selective, undermining, and destructive, as within subgroups, for example. Sometimes we even "subgroup" with ourselves—originating and validating negative internal dialogues that stalemate our communication's effectiveness. So, when we talk about having open, honest communications, we must first learn to control the dialogue within ourselves. When our whole team is in integrity, it is awesome and powerful.

This leads to the fourth aspect of the context — relationships. When there is a shared vision, supportive agreements, and open communication, relationships form naturally. These relationships are emotionally rewarding, and work becomes an enjoyable part of life.

Now that we have the four ingredients for the context of our team in place, we can look at distinctions of outstanding, long-term teams. These teams are connected, integrated, and powerful. They stand the test of time because they have key elements in place.

First, there must be *source* people in your practice. The source is simply the person accountable for the result. This person may have nothing to do with the *doing* of a project or department, however, they are accountable that the tasks are completed.

Competent source people must oversee several areas of the dental practice. We can take our model from corporate America and look at our dental practices.

There are three distinct departments in our practice – Operative, Hygiene, and Business Administration. There are also three accelerators in our practice that provide the patient flow that we need to maintain our daily schedules – marketing (new patients), hygiene reactivation, and treatment reactivation.

Creating accountability provides structure and a context in which to manage the most critical aspects of our practice. Let me ask you a question. In corporate America, if the janitor ran out of toilet paper supplies, do you think he would go to the CEO to get more? Absolutely not! Does this happen in our dental practices? You bet, at least it did in my office. Wouldn't it make more sense to keep the doctor's hands on the hand piece? What would happen to our productivity if the doctor was focused on the clinical aspects of the practice and not on the toilet paper?

In a multi-doctor practice, I recommend that we still have one primary source doctor and the other doctors take on supporting coaching roles. For example, one doctor could be the primary source for the clinical staff, while another could be the source for the marketing and administrative aspects of the practice.

If each person stays on track as a source person, then what happens to your practice? Each department stays on track, the marketing, re-care and reactivation activities stay on track. Our practices stay on track!

The second quality of outstanding teams is integrity. Most people equate integrity with honesty. If you look integrity up in the dictionary, honesty is actually about number four or five in the definition. The primary definition is completeness or wholeness. Recalling our analogy of your team as a glass of water, if we don't have completeness or wholeness in our glass, then the integrity is impaired. You begin to lose content due to the lack of integrity in the glass. For example:

As I was traveling to deliver an in-office consultation, I was met at the airport by a hygienist. When I got into her car, what can you imagine I found between the seat and the door jam? A fossilized hamburger wedged by the edge of the seat! It was not only disgusting, but it gave me insight into her personal standards as well as the degree of integrity that she stood for in the practice.

I'd like to offer this philosophy to you. The degree to which we are out of integrity in one part of our life, subconsciously becomes the degree to which it is acceptable in every area of our life. So, when there is a little bit of mess in our car, then its okay in our house, then its okay in the appointment book, or on our monitors. Can you see how this can quickly impact the quality of your practice?

We are only as strong as our weakest link. I see it on a daily basis in the outstanding teams that I work with. Top performance teams are impeccable in their commitment to maintaining integrity in their practices. This includes upholding the vision statement and all the agreements that support it, particularly the agreements concerning communication, patient interaction, and long-term financial success of the practice. Whenever someone is out of integrity with his commitments, then a source person coaches him back in place. If it is a source person who needs coaching, then anyone on the team who sees the breach is at liberty to coach the situation. High level, outstanding teams become very protective of their environment and will not allow substandard behavior to infiltrate their structure.

The third quality of outstanding teams is safety. What I am referring to here is the ability for people to freely express their ideas, concerns, and suggestions. Staff members need to know that they have permission to communicate appropriately their needs without fear of retribution or dismissal. The doctor also needs to know that it is safe to communicate with the staff, in an appropriate manner, and know that people will not resign from the practice as a result. When we allow this type of free flow of ideas we have the ability to quickly remove frustrations from our daily routine. This is a critical achievement skill as we move into an era that demands quick decision and the ability to be flexible in our approach to patient care.

If this level of safety is not present for your practice, who is responsible for creating this safety? You are! Invest in your staff. Every member of your team should be trained in communication technology that will enhance the relationships of the practice. Each practice should have *states people* who assist in facilitating this process. The *states person* is simply someone committed to safe, open, honest communications in the practice, and willing to be held accountable for relationships staying on track.

The fourth quality of outstanding teams is coaching. As a coach, you must be willing not to have the answers. Your position is one of questioning, finding out what is working, and what is not working. Acknowledge those who have contributed, recommit to the result, and make declarations and requests of your teammates.

As a coach to dental practices for more than 15 years, I have used this basic formula time and time again, with remarkable results. What I have found in life is that the answer always lies in the question.

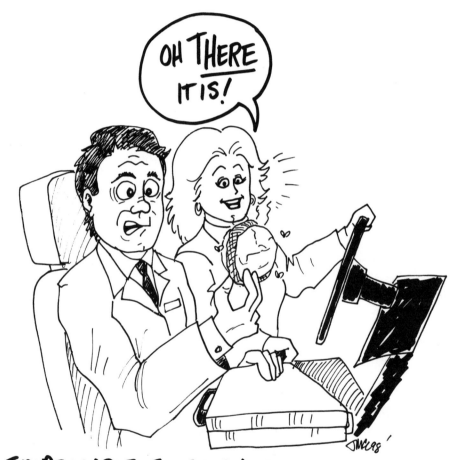

Creating Your Vision

In an uninterrupted environment, take time to relax and ask yourself the following questions. Start with a blank sheet of paper or flipchart, and write down whatever comes to mind.

List all the emotions you want to experience on a consistent basis.

List the feelings that you want to evoke in others that you have contact with (staff and patients.)

Use descriptive words to describe your desired professional reputation, or what you want to be known for in your community.

Use short phrases, or words to describe where you "see" your practice in five years?

It is important that you NOT analyze your responses to these questions. Just write down whatever comes to mind; your vision is something that has not taken place yet! Take a moment to look at your lists and then use this sample format to construct your personal vision statement.

As a _____ (describe the type of practice-remember to use adjectives) with a reputation for _____, we are committed to _____ (service or feelings you provide). It is our purpose to support _____ (describe the ways you support each other and your patients.)

Example:

As a dynamic, growing practice with an international reputation for state of the art excellence, we are committed to providing impeccable dentistry by an educated, passionate, and motivated team, which supports personal creativity and growth in an exemplary work place.

Creating Supportive Agreements

Using the example above, here are a few sample agreements that would need to be in place to support this vision and make it a reality.

I agree to support the policies and agreements of this practice, coming from a place of honesty and integrity.

I agree to support others in keeping their agreements.

I agree to be on time for workdays, and to stay to completion of each day.

If I am unable to attend a workday, I will contact the Doctor at the first possible moment, and replace myself for that day.

I agree to participate 100% in staff meetings, and continuing education.

As a healthcare professional, I understand that I am responsible for my own health and well being; I will present myself every day in the physical condition necessary to work within this practice: well-rested, alert, and properly nourished.

I agree to accept responsibility for my actions, and to create an environment whereby co-workers feel safe to express themselves through open, honest communication.

I agree to handle any complaints that I may have by communicating them only to the person who can do something about the situation. I further agree not to criticize or complain to someone who cannot do anything about the situation. I agree not to receive, from anyone, complaints that I cannot do something about; but rather agree to redirect that person to someone who can do something about it.

These are just a few agreements that may need to be in place in order to support the vision of having a *"dynamic, growing practice… committed to providing impeccable dentistry by an educated, passionate and motivated team… which supports personal creativity and growth in an exemplary workplace."*

As a team, mastermind agreements that you need to have to make your vision a reality. Remember: Agreements are NOT rules — they are a code of conduct that everyone shares. This is the basis of accountability in your practice.

A. Paul Bass, III, D.D.S.

Is cofounder and Chairman of Fortune Practice Management® — an Anthony Robbins Company, based in San Diego, CA. He received his D.D.S. degree from the University of Tennessee in 1972 and practiced clinically for more than 20 years. He and his wife Lyn, enjoy the company of their three daughters.

For the past fifteen years, Dr. Bass has been a perpetual student of personal growth and development, with a specific focus on team building and motivation. He has presented over 2,500 seminars, workshops, and training programs that have positively impacted tens of thousands of people.

Dr. Bass is the creator of the audio cassette series Practice Mastery, which emphasizes team building skills. For information regarding Dr. Bass' seminars or cassette programs call (800) 687-3393 or Fax (931) 455-0522 or E-mail: FPMMIDTN@compuserve.com

Words of Wisdom 🦷

I feel it is very important to treat all staff members equally. I do not give special favors to clinical staff or business staff. All staff members arrive at the same time and leave at the same time. If one staff member is finished with her patients, she helps the other staff members.

DR. KIMBERLY A. CARVER-HARPER
Warner Robbins, GA

The patients are our priority. We are all employees, all equals. If we all do our jobs, we all benefit… I don't put myself on a pedestal — I will clean rooms, vacuum, pull charts, answer the phone, schedule appointments, etc.

DR. DEBBY MATTHEWS
Lafayette, LA

We train each person extensively to be a leader. We train each one to run the practice.

DR. OWEN JUSTICE
Las Vegas, NV

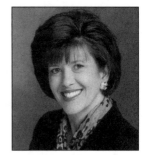

Chapter Six

The 'Root' of Team Development: Understanding the Stages of Team Building

Vicki McManus, RDH

"If it's not FUN, you're not doing it right." — Bob Basso

As a consultant, I am frequently challenged to find out what teams really need and as a result have discovered a common theme among dental practices. "We want cooperative, motivated staff, with outstanding emotional and financial rewards, and we want them NOW." Is this statement true for you? If so, then learning what I have termed the FASTR™ cycle of team building will be a powerful tool in your practice. FASTR™ stands for the five stages of team building: Formation, Adjustment, Stabilization, Top Performance, and Restoration.

The FASTR™ model is based on the work of many psychologists and experts in human interaction. Researching this book, I found that most models for team building come from either athletic or corporate perspectives and describe four stages of team building, most popularly known as *forming, storming, norming,* and *performing.* Most team building models have limited application to dentistry because they don't encompass the longevity of our dental teams. Ideally, wouldn't you like to reduce staff turnover and create teams that surpass the national average tenure of 3.5 years? With this thought, I added a fifth stage — Restoration, as a recognized stage of team building to describe the repetitive nature of the first four stages.

As you learn about the stages of team building and relate them to your practice, there are several key concepts to bear in mind.

- Each stage is a necessary aspect of your growth.
- You can't move to the next level until you master the level you are in.
- The feelings that you are experiencing in each stage are *natural* responses to your circumstances. It does no good to dismiss, deny, defend or justify them.
- Each time a change occurs in your practice, you will begin reforming your team on some level. Your challenge is to recognize this and restore the balance as quickly as possible.
- We are focused 100% on patient care only in the Top Performance level. All other stages divert our focus elsewhere in the practice.
- "There is no 'I' in TEAM" is a myth. Every Individual plays an important part; don't diminish the impact (positive and negative) that you have on your TEAM.
- There are no *born leaders*. Leadership is a learned skill.

Stage One: Formation

It's the bottom of the ninth with three men on base and two outs. The score is tied. The batter steps up to the plate. With a count of three and two, he swings — connects. It's out of here! IT'S A GRAND SLAM HOME RUN! Our hometown boys have done it again! The crowd goes wild.

This is the image of a winning team. For years you have stood to cheer the victories of others, but now it's time to form your own winning team. The first step is to create a conscious bond using three essential elements: leadership, shared vision, and common communication.

In the early *formation* period, potential team members are not sure what to expect. Here's the doctor's opportunity/responsibility to relieve confusion or anxiety by clearly defining the goals of his practice and by integrating future team members in a positive, productive manner.

Team members form first and sometimes permanent impressions noting similarities, and in this stage in particular, differences. Each member works on issues of inclusion and decides to join the team or not. Some questions influencing decisions are:

- Is the doctor a competent leader?
- Do I like his/her style of leadership?
- Do I want to be a part of this team?
- Will I be accepted as a team member?
- How will I interact with others?

Because of confusion or anxiety in the early stages of team building, there is a tendency for the team to rely heavily on the leadership of the doctor. This is especially true, since it is the doctor's vision that molds the practice. With the assistance of a facilitator or coach, this vision is shared, integrated, and revised when necessary.

Stage Two: Adjustment

Draft picks have been made. The new team is ready for spring training; but, as you board the bus for Florida, you notice two of your players in a petty argument. What is going on? You haven't even had a chance to play together and the "artistic differences" have already taken the field. Welcome to the second stage of team building — *adjustment*.

Characterized by competition and strained relationships, the adjustment stage deals with power, leadership, and decision-making. During this most critical stage, team members often recognize the discrepancy between the *vision* and the daily reality. Some team members will openly question the wisdom of their leaders — doctor, office manager, and/or consultant/coach of the practice. In order to assert their individuality and influence, they may also resist efforts to define their tasks.

Because it is human nature to *circle the wagons* during times of conflict, team members may self-servingly deny the contributions of others and resort to other non-supportive behaviors such as: uniting in counterproductive subgroups, being late, missing meetings, adopting a TNMJ (that's not my job) attitude.

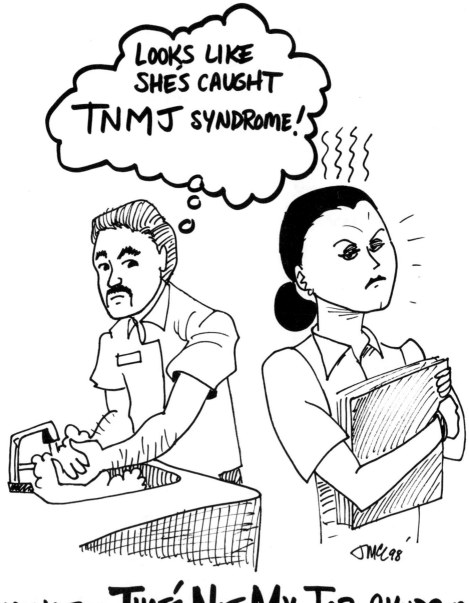

Each member is addressing the issue of control and determining whether it is safe to be a member of the team. Some questions raised during this phase are:

- How will I seek my autonomy?
- How much influence do I have in this team?
- How much control will I have over others?
- How much control will others try to have over me?
- Whom do I support?
- Who supports me?

The team must work through this conflict stage, or it will find itself unable to develop into a fully functioning team, much less the team of the original vision. Here is where most staff turnover in dentistry occurs, and thus the team will continue to cycle back through the forming stage until it resolves both professional and personal issues.

Stage Three: Stabilization

The first ray of sun has peeked through after a night of storming weather. You open your eyes to see a rainbow in the distance. All is right with the world and your new team is adjusting nicely. They are forming good relationships and addressing concerns in a productive manner. This is the stabilization stage of team development, which is characterized by a growing cohesiveness among team members. After working through the adjustment period, members find that they do, in fact, have common interests. While still learning to appreciate their differences, they feel more harmonious as a team and begin to problem solve together.

At this point, the team starts to become a cohesive unit. The key word is "starts" because they will still attempt to renegotiate their roles and tasks. However, team members are now committed to working with the others. Functional relationships have developed and leadership issues are resolved through cooperative, interdependent behavior. As the most essential element of teams, *trust* emerges, the team grows in solidarity. Questions that are raised in this stage of development include:

- What kind of relationship can we develop?
- What is my relationship to the team leader?
- Will we be successful as a team?
- How do we measure up to other teams?

And so the turmoil of the *adjustment stage* has been relieved by a heightened sense of belonging. The animosity towards the leader and other team members has diminished to normal, healthy interpersonal relationships. The key is to nurture trust and rapport among team members. Talk openly about issues and concerns.

Stage Four: Top Performance

"Popcorn, peanuts, get your ice-cold cola!" It's game time. You've finally made it past spring training. Your team is out of the dugout, in position on the playing field and ready to perform. The stage of *top performance* is the culmination of the first three stages.

Team members are aware of and accountable for their tasks. By this stage, they have learned to work together as a fully functioning team — defining tasks, managing conflicts, enjoying relationships, achieving goals, even realizing the vision. Leadership is shared and participatory. All this without fear of rejection because communication is open, supportive, and hence creative. This is the most harmonious stage — Congratulations! You're winning the game.

Stage Five: Restoration

... And they never lost a game.

You've just developed your new team. Members have weathered the storms and the type of cooperation you have always dreamed of exists in your practice. There will never be another "slump" for your team. Right? Wrong. Unfortunately, any change in team dynamics can cause a team to revisit the developmental cycle.

Changes in team dynamics can include any changes in the structure of the team. Hiring additional or replacing existing staff, or transitioning an associate doctor will definitely cause recycling. Likewise, changes in physical structure of the practice or implementation of new technology can also upset the balance of the team. Events like holidays, weddings, divorce, or children leaving for college can trigger regression of the team. Even team accomplishment can lead to a "let down" effect and cause temporary regression. Consider the following scenario.

You've just had your best month ever. Production, collections, and the number of new patients are up. Everyone seems happy — Until. Until, your first staff meeting. Goals or a mission statement are brought to the table. Someone suggests that you could stretch and accomplish even more while someone else questions *why*? Resistance builds. Some members become quiet and withdrawn leaving room for the vocal few. The team has been transported back to the adjustment stage once again! How do you quickly move through this adjustment phase and regain your strength as a *top performance team*?

Questions concerning the purpose of growth, stretching the team mission or goals demands heightened awareness. Make sure that you ask questions such as:

- How can we grow in a way that is consistent with our values?
- What would happen if we didn't put a limit on our capacity?
- How can we support each other in this growth process?

Since you know that it is possible to experience temporary setbacks in your team, even after periods of success, you can prepare ahead of time. Become a master of the team's language, looking for signs such as doubt, negative attitudes, or slight resistance that indicate a reversion to an earlier stage. Track your progress through the month, reinforce team accomplishments, share pride in their hard work, and include staff in masterminding ways to maintain the momentum. Ask them to be conscious of thoughts and words, which might have a negative effect on the team. Let's review the questions frequently asked during the formation, adjustment and stabilization stages of team building:

- What price will I pay to belong to this team?
- How much control will I have over others?
- How much control will others try to have over me?
- How much influence do I have in this team?
- Is the leader competent?

Our goal is to create self-authorized team leaders who accept accountability for the practice. With the complexities facing dentistry today, it is impossible for the doctor to handle the entire management burden. He/she must have team members who function in an open, honest, synergistic manner. Understanding the stages of team building is the center piece of the puzzle.

To have fully engaged team members requires recognition of each member's current status as well as scouting for what is needed to enhance their self-esteem and security. For instance, Xerox recently conducted a personnel study and concluded that 70% of all peak performers leave their jobs because they don't feel they can express their thoughts and ideas. I suspect the same is true in dentistry.

You have been given valuable tools to utilize throughout the various stages of team building. Most books written on the subject stop after the performance cycle which is analogous to the ending of most Disney movies. Whatever happened to Cinderella and Prince Charming?

Creating an environment of "win – win – win" whereby the owner/leaders win, the staff wins, your referral network wins, and the patient wins, is what I term, the *connective advantage.* This type of synergy breaks the paycheck mentality and allows staff to gain psychological ownership of the practice.

Effective daily performance and commitment are tested and sustained by understanding each other's feelings and personal objectives. I've included exercises for your team to work through twice per year. Complete them now and mark your calendar to repeat in six months. The purpose is to open communications and to clarify objectives of individual team members.

Team Commitment Exercise

Good for Me Checklist

from Section II, Games to Help Teams Function

Objective: To provide each team member with a self-administered assessment tally that functions as a behavior modification tool as team members learn to work together as a team.

Procedure: Give each team member a GOOD FOR ME CHECKLIST
               to be used to record individuals' good team behaviors each
               day for one week. Repeat the exercise as many weeks as you
               need to as team members get used to team behavior.

               Hand this out perhaps on a Friday, near the end of a team
               meeting or training session, for a Monday morning start. The
               benefits from this checklist are largely for the individual
               who fills it out, but the completed checklist can also be used
               as a foundation for a team meeting or discussion between a
               team member and a supervisor or team leader.

               Suggest to trainees that these are some "good for me"
               behaviors they should try out: identify a problem, identify a
               solution, verbally support another's effective actions, deal
               directly with someone who can fix a problem, share feelings
               with another, meet or exceed a standard, manage conflict,
               clarify something, share control, share leadership, accept
               criticism, act on feedback from someone, give constructive
               feedback.

Discussion
Questions: Ask trainees to pay special attention to the people whom
               they have helped, the people who made their own good
               actions possible, the systems support that they got or the
               systems that their actions improved, the procedures that they
               they fixed, or the tasks that they performed with greater skill
               or impact.

               Ask trainees to be aware of quality in both the content and
               the processes of their jobs during the week.

A new team member is faced with the monumental task of
changing his or her thinking and way of doing work so that
relationships, processes, and systems become more important
than individually pleasing one's boss, isolated tasks, and
narrowly defined job functions. People need to be encouraged
to maintain their own personal integrity and standards of
performance quality as they move toward excellence as a
contributor to the team. This behavior modification tool can
help individuals in this transition.

Materials: A GOOD FOR ME CHECKLIST for each trainee

Approximate
Time Required: One week of lapse time; several minutes each day

GOOD FOR ME CHECKLIST

During the week, try to become aware of exactly what you are doing to make the team work better. Use this GOOD FOR ME CHECKLIST to reward yourself for each specific good behavior. Give yourself a check mark every time you do something important to make the team function better. Do this every day for one week, taking a few minutes to take stock of your actions before lunch and before leaving for home at the end of the day. Accompany each check marke with a brief note about what you did. Add more items and more pages as appropriate, with check marks in the appropriate columns.

	M	Tu	W	Th	F	Notes
1. Asked for help						
2. Took criticism						
3. Provided feedback						
4. Identified a problem						
5. Solved a problem						
6. Increased my skill level						
7. Supported a team member						
8. Accepted leadership						
9. Gave up leadership						
10. Complimented another's work						
11. Facilitated a decision						
12. Called a meeting						

Sweet Success

Objective: To encourage team members to analyze their work situations and identify areas for improvement. The goal is for the team leader's jar to be full of a variety of jelly beans and for each team member to have contributed approximately the same number of jelly beans at the end of the play period.

Procedure: This game is a variation of the suggestion box. A time limit, such as a specific week of each month for the next six months, is designated. During this time, team members are asked to focus on finding work processes, situations, or procedures that are problems impeding the building of the team. You may also include suggestions for improving patient experiences with your office.

As each person finds a problem, he/she takes one jelly bean from his/her jar, writes the problem on the "problem sign-in sheet" and places the jelly bean in the team leader's jar.

The team leader should keep a clipboard with a "problem sign-in sheet" next to his/her desk next to the candy jar. The top of the sheet should read:

"What's Your Sweet Problem Today?"

At the end of each agreed-upon time for playing the game, time should be allocated during your weekly staff meeting to have a general discussion about the nature of the problems identified on the list.

Remember: This is an exercise in problem identification, *not* problem solutions. Keep the discussion general and identify areas that you would like to work on. Place that item on the next agenda, ask for a volunteer to source the project, create a game plan, or take other appropriate action to begin the solution process.

Materials: One large jelly bean container (preferably glass for the leader); one jelly bean jar and one single color bag of jelly beans for each team member.

Time Required: Several minutes per day, 10 — 15 minutes in staff meeting.

Reward: Everyone gets to eat the jelly beans at the staff meeting!!! And celebrate the ideas and suggestions that are put forth. Remember every team member's opinion is valid and necessary for growth.

Bean Counter Problem Sign-In Sheet

What's Your Sweet Problem Today?

Date	Time	Sweet Problem	Initials

© 1993, McGraw-Hill, Nilson, C. and Philip Ruppel, <u>Team Games for Trainers</u>.

Please print. Limit your responses to one line per suggestion. Thank you for your commitment to the growth of this team.

Vicki McManus, RDH

Since 1979 Vicki has been a part of the solution for the challenges facing dentistry and dental hygiene. A practicing clinical hygienist for 15 years, she now empowers others to create success strategies in both their personal and professional lives.

Vicki is the founder of the Lifetime Learning Center — a company dedicated to lifelong learning and development. As cofounder of Creative Excellence, Inc. and Director of Fortune Practice Management® — Connecticut, she coaches healthcare teams to decrease stress and increase profitability through teamwork.

She holds memberships in the Institute of Management Consultants, National Speakers Association, Candidate Member — Institute of Certified Financial Planners, and the American Dental Hygienists Association. She is actively involved in speaking and presenting throughout the United States and Canada.

For more information on her interactive seminar programs "Team Building is FUNdamental™" or "Building a Healthy Hygiene Department" or you want to receive her Fax newsletter called FUNdamentals™ of Outstanding Dental Teams, call (888) 347-4785, Fax (770) 512-0892 or E-mail FPMVicki@compuserve.com

Words of Wisdom

In our office we rotate the staff members as leaders of our monthly staff meetings. This gives them responsibility [for various tasks].
DR. TIMOTHY JON CLAY & DR. ROSEMARY CLAY
Wilmington, DE

The doctor must be the example. The head leads — the body follows. Our excellent team is synchronized and focused on constant improvement to achieve a common goal: To deliver excellence in dental service with compassion for every patient's need.
DR. SUE WEISHAAR
Spokane, WA

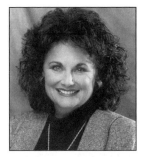

Chapter Seven

Tell the 'Tooth, the Whole Tooth': Great Communication — The Bottom Line to Successful Teamwork

Cathy Jameson, M.A.

"The quality of your life depends on the quality of your communication. To get a better result ask a better question." — ANTHONY ROBBINS

The team is the *lifeblood* and the *heartbeat* of the dental practice. My definition of a great dental team is "a group of leaders focusing on a common set of goals." When the time, talent, and potential of the individual members of the organization are focused on those goals, energy converges and productivity increases.

Effective communication is a critical element of successful teamwork. Without it teams experience dysfunction, turnover, low energy, and decreased productivity. Thus, an ongoing study of communication will be emotionally, physically, and financially beneficial to all — the doctor, the team members, and the practice.

Have you ever been involved in a conversation with a co-worker and felt as if you were on "am" and they were on "fm?" The reality may have been that you were in total agreement with one another; but because of the language that you were using — your thoughts were not clearly conveyed or received.

Let's study aspects of communication: listening, speaking, and problem solving.

Listening

Lee Iacocca believes that "listening can make the difference between a mediocre company and a good company." Sperry, one of America's major companies, values the skill of listening so highly that it has courses on listening available to all levels of personnel. Sperry believes that the inability to listen leads to such business inefficiencies as:

- wasted time
- inefficient operation of departments
- miscarried plans
- frustrated decisions in every phase of the business

And so, good companies need good teamwork, and good teamwork needs good listening. In fact, most people agree that, while good listening is invaluable, it is most often an ideal and not the reality. As Kevin Murphy puts it in Effective Listening "Listening is a natural process that goes against human nature." What gets in the way of good listening in the dental environment?

- time pressure
- stress — not being relaxed
- mind set — being rigid in thought process
- talking too much — dominating the conversation as the authority
- thinking of what to say in response instead of listening lack of interest
- ego — "I know the answer" or "I know what to do, so I don't need to listen to you."

Four Aspects of Listening

1. Body Language

Approximately 60% of the perception of a message — whether it is being sent or received—depends on the body language. You can make or break a conversation by your body language. Even though the words may be just right, the message can be misinterpreted if the body language delivers a mixed message.

Positive body language expressions include: establishing and maintaining eye contact, being on the same physical level, touching, nodding or shaking the head, facial expression, reflecting the other person's body movements, and having an open stance.

Paying attention to body language is vital to communication. If 60% of the perception of the message is related to body language, it makes good sense to be ever aware of how you are coming across to another person—particularly if you want the other person to sense that you are, indeed, listening.

2. Tone of Voice

Paul Harvey says, "It's not what you say, it's how you say it." The way a person delivers a message can alter the entire reception. Tone of voice accounts for approximately 30% of the perception of a message. Add the 30% tone of voice to the 60% body language and you can easily see that even though your words can be terrific, the meaning of your words can be altered significantly if the body language and the tone of voice do not complement the message.

You must be the one who is flexible adopting a tone of voice congruent to the content of the message. If you want to convey a caring, receptive attitude, soften your voice; if authority is the emphasis, strengthen it. If you are with a high energy, fast-talker — speed it up; or adjust accordingly to someone with a more slow, deliberate style. This reflection of the other person will increase his comfort and encourage his sharing.

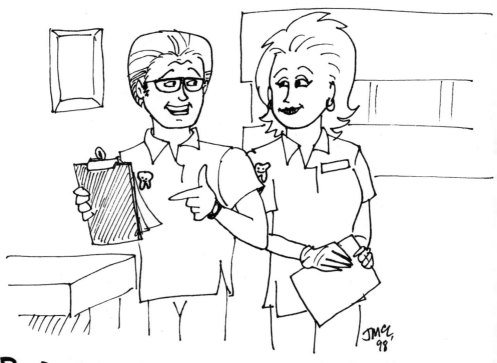

BE DIRECT WITH YOUR COMMUNICATIONS!

3. Passive Listening

Often a person expressing a concern or problem isn't asking for advice but for attention and care. Non-supportive response, such as giving advice prematurely, or being overly critical can build barriers to communication, effectively closing the doors to further communication. When a person begins telling you something, you need as much information as possible. Information lets you identify motivators, problems, concerns, and emotions.

By practicing excellent listening, you allow another person to deal with his own issues. You allow him to clarify, not only to you but to himself, some of the questions that may exist. No one can solve a problem for a person except that person. Listening helps to define the problem so that successful problem solving can take place.

Don't take away from a person's ability to deal with his own issues. Be an enhancer. Listen. Listen without judgment. Allow a person to have separate feelings from you and to deal with them. Know that if a person wants your opinion, he will ask for it.

Be attentive, passive listening encourages a person to get it all out. Ask a question and then respond with a non-stimulating response. Passive listening means you are hearing what the other person is saying, but you are careful not to interfere with the commentary. Passive listening responses might be: "I see." "I understand." "Uh, huh." "Continue." 'Hmmm." "Tell me more." "I agree."

Use excellent body language; respond with passive listening messages; let the other person continue without interruption. Don't try to fill all silent moments. Silence is full of messages and gives time to organize thoughts, gain the confidence to go on, and express deeper feelings.

The most challenging part of passive listening is asking the question and then waiting for the person to respond without interrupting!! When you ask that question — **BE QUIET!** Let him answer — even if a few moments of silence occurs.

4. Active Listening

The single most effective listening skill you can use to calm an irate person, to defuse anger, to handle a difficult person, or on the other hand — to enhance a good relationship — is to listen actively. This kind of listening requires effort and discipline.

Active listening is feeding back to people what you think you have heard them saying to make sure that you have heard them correctly. A simple repetition or paraphrasing is not sufficient. The listener should demonstrate, in his/her own words, an adequate understanding of the content, intent, and emotion of the speaker's remarks.

This type of listening lets you clarify to make sure that you understand what the person is trying to say. Active listening is used when someone comes to you with a problem or a concern. The other person owns the problem.

Examples:
1) Team member — "Sarah makes so many mistakes. She's driving me crazy."
Office Manager — "You seem frustrated by Sarah's performance these days."
2) Assistant — "I'm not sure I'm ready to assist you with that procedure yet."
Doctor — "Sounds like you're feeling uncomfortable because you're unsure of how to perform this new technique."

With active listening, the problem isn't solved — it's identified. Once it is identified, then a problem-solving scenario can begin. Too many people wrap solutions around problems and never take the time to identify the true problem.

One of the main purposes of active listening is to keep misunderstandings to a minimum. When you are involved in a listening situation, make sure that you do so with sincerity, understanding, acceptance, and caring. Listen to your teammates. *Open Doors.*

The Communication Flow

Excellent communication takes place when the message sent by the speaker is interpreted correctly by the listener. Obviously, both of the skills — listening and speaking — are critical for the communication flow to work.

Speaking so that others will listen and understand is one part of the communication flow. All members of your team have the opportunity to move a relationship further along — or to pull that relationship to a stop by the way they communicate. The goals of good speaking are the following:

- To help people *want* to listen to what you have to say.
- To deliver the message in the best possible manner.
- To check to see if you were heard (or interpreted) correctly.

There's the goal — to have communication experiences become a mutual involvement of all parties — to have interactions that encourage the giving and receiving of information and feelings. Result? Winning relationships. Strong relationships.

The Flow of Communication

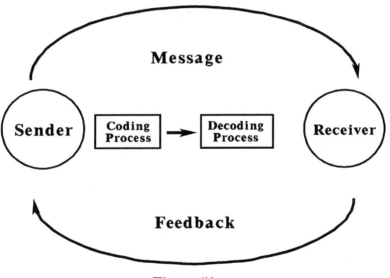

Figure #1

Sending Clear Messages

Effective communication takes place (as illustrated in Figure #1) when there is a clear sending of a message (speaking skills) and appropriate feedback to check the accuracy of the reception (listening skills). In other words, "Did you get my message?" and "Am I hearing you right?" It is definitely a two-way process.

A person sends a message either verbally or nonverbally — or both. The information that the speaker wants to convey to the receiver is transformed into outward behavior (verbal or nonverbal.)

The message is received by the other person who then interprets the message based on prior experience and understanding. Feelings are produced in reaction to the interpretation, and judgments are made about the intention of the message.

Receiving or requesting feedback gives the sender of the message a chance to know if the message has been heard accurately — or if it needs to be clarified. This feedback may be the best communicative skill you can ever access — the skill of determining if your message has been sent and received accurately.

Addressing Challenging Issues

You have learned the skills of listening so that you can be more helpful and you have learned speaking skills to deliver your message more clearly. However, you may now be asking yourself: "Great! I know what to do to help others if they have a problem. I know how to speak effectively, but what do I do when I have a *problem* with someone, and I want to get my message across or I need help?"

If someone's behavior is having *a concrete (definable) negative effect on you, on your performance, or on the practice,* then you have not only the right but also the responsibility to address the issue. It's imperative that you address the behavior and not the person. It's important to let a person know that you may not like his behavior but that you still like him.

Some people have a difficult time hearing about their own behavior. They take constructive criticism personally and become offended by the confrontation. Therefore, learning to speak in a nonthreatening manner will move you closer to the goal of being able to confront constructively — not harmfully.

Nevertheless, you need and deserve to have your needs met. In order to be successful in getting your needs met, certain speaking skills are necessary — and beneficial. Developing excellent speaking skills will accomplish the following goals:

- let you get your message across accurately
- have your needs understood and met
- move your relationships to the next level
- to gain a person's trust and confidence

"I" Messages

In <u>Leadership Effectiveness Training,</u> Dr. Thomas Gordon suggests that when you own a problem — that is, when someone is having a concrete negative effect on you, on your performance, or on the practice — you need to confront that person. People are often reluctant to confront because of fear of hurting or angering the other person, but not confronting someone whose behavior is causing a problem doesn't serve either party well. If a person is unaware that what he is doing is inappropriate, he can't change; and, overall, the problem escalates.

Essential to constructive confrontation is the "I" message. The "I" message is not the problem solver, but it is an excellent way to get the problem defined or clarified. That is the first step in problem solving — to define the problem. An "I" message is a clear, accurate code sent when someone is causing you a problem. It is a message made up of three specific parts:

1. The sincere emotion you are feeling.
2. A brief description of the behavior you find unacceptable.
3. The concrete, negative effect or result of that behavior.

A sample format for an "I" message is as follows:

I feel _____
                                 (sincere emotion)

when _____
                              (unacceptable behavior)

because _____.
                              (concrete, negative result)

Example:

"I am feeling concerned that we are having so many no shows and broken appointments. This causes a lot of stress for everyone — including you, of course."

This type of careful communication expresses your particular problem in a nonthreatening, nonjudgmental manner. More than likely, the person will not become angry but will see your side and be willing to work things out.

You Message

The opposite of an "I" message is a "You" message — or a put-down message — in which blame, judgment, and intimidation are the net result of the statement. Most people are great at sending "You" messages. This type of message causes defensive or antagonistic responses.

Example:

"You aren't getting the patients scheduled well enough. You don't do a good job of confirming, and we are having too many broken appointments and no shows. You had better clean up your act."

Problem Solving

Once a problem has been identified through effective listening and "I" messages, move into a problem-solving scenario. The following is a synopsis of problem solving — a process that will work for you if it is followed with commitment.

1. Identify the problem in terms of the needs of each party.
2. Brainstorm possible solutions.
3. Discuss each possible solution.
4. Come to a consensus decision about which solution or solutions will work best.
5. Design a plan of action — who will do what by when.
6. Implement the plan.
7. Get back together on a regular basis to see if things are working. In other words, evaluate.

Great communication equals great production. Cohesive team members listen to each other with respect and when a conflict arises, they address the issue head on with careful and constructive confrontation. If the team members — either individually or as a group — focus on problem solving — whether the problem is major or minor, great teamwork will become a reality for you.

Activity

List three frustrations or challenges that you have with someone on your team. Determine if their behavior is having a concrete, negative effect on you or your practice. If so, work through the "I" message format to communicate your needs to this person. If their behavior is not having a concrete, negative effect on you or your team, then let go of the frustration and celebrate the stress relief!

Frustration/Challenge that needs to be Communicated

1. _____
   concrete, negative effect?   _____yes _____no
2. _____
   concrete, negative effect?   _____yes _____no
3. _____
   concrete, negative effect?   _____yes _____no

Communication Process

_____ (person with whom you are upset)
I feel _____ (sincere emotion)
when _____ (unacceptable behavior)
because _____ (concrete, negative result)
I need your help in resolving this issue.

Use listening skills to activate problem-solving process. Continue opening lines of communication until workable solution is achieved.

Cathy Jameson, B.S., M.A.

Cathy is the President of Jameson Management Group and Dental Advantage Consulting, an international dental consulting firm. An accomplished speaker, writer and workshop leader, Cathy holds a bachelor's degree in education and a master's degree in psychology. As a certified Effectiveness Trainer, Cathy integrates her academic background and her knowledge of communication into the management of dental teams and practices. Her 25 years of hands on experience in the practice of her dentist husband, Dr. John H. Jameson, make her strategies workable and effective.

She has been a featured speaker for the major dental meetings throughout the world and is also an adjunct faculty member of the Oklahoma University School of Dentistry. Cathy's books, Great Communication = Great Production and Collect what you Produce are top sellers in the dental arena for PennWell Books. For more information call (580) 369-5555 or (580) 369-2501.

Words of Wisdom 🦷

All team members are encouraged to openly exchange any ideas that will improve overall performance or attitude of the team. This applies whether it affects them directly or indirectly and does not have to be formally expressed at our morning huddle.

DR. DENNIS LIND
Buffalo Grove, IL

When team members go to continuing education courses, they discuss their findings with the other staff and me.

DR. RANDAL BOURJAILY
Novi, MI

Everyone wears jeans and a sweatshirt, and we have a large trash bag which we throw out everything in the office we no longer need. We then try to guess what certain items are!! We then order a pizza and laugh about our "pack rat habits" and the stupid things we bought and didn't need.

DR. WILLIAM OAKES
New Albany, IN

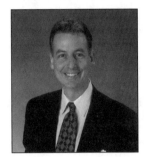

Chapter Eight

Staff Meetings that 'Bond': Guaranteeing Productive Staff Meetings

Doug Smart

"The best meetings grab hold of possibility thinking and ignite brain power!" — DOUG SMART

True or false? 80% of all meetings you have attended in your professional life were a *colossal waste of your time!* True for me, and I bet true for you. Once, in a large organization, my job description tangled me in a net that snagged all the decision-makers into the biweekly Thursday afternoon three-hour managers' meeting marathon. Mr. Number 1 (the owner of the company) rarely attended because, he said, he couldn't spare the time. So, Mr. Number 2 (the aspiring executive) administered the meeting: "…good work, Mary. Now, Doug, bring us up to date on what's going on in *your* department… Good job, Doug. Next, it looks like, Jerry, it's your turn…" The chairs were leather, the table marble, and the art work lit by tiny museum spotlights; my numbed mind, however, plopped me behind a little wooden desk in third grade struggling to keep my eyes open through afternoon book reports. As my business brain cells surfaced for oxygen, I thought of the things I would rather be working on and the cost to the business to bring us together.

What are *your* meetings like? Are they healthy exchanges of information best delivered face-to-face? Do they extinguish conflicts? Do they inspire fresh new solutions to surprising new challenges? How do the patients benefit from your office meetings? Do your meetings get you closer to achieving your short and long-term goals? What is the impact on the bottom line? In this chapter we will look at why you need to meet, different types of meetings to accomplish this "why," ground rules for great meetings, and some fun ways to spark ideas for improving patient care, office operation, and a healthier bottom line.

Why Meet?

To succeed, we need each other. Meetings are a medium of communication. On the surface, we communicate information needed to operate the office effectively; but, at a deeper level, we absorb information from each other that nourishes our intra-office relationships. We need both. In one of my seminars, a doctor told me she has a meeting with her office manager every Friday afternoon from 5:30 to 6. It's just the two of them. They schedule so that there aren't any patients at that time, they are unavailable by phone (as reasonably as they can), and they will not catch up on paperwork. They own those thirty minutes, during which they discuss the events of the past week and the events of the week coming up. Do you think these two people have a mature working relationship? Do you think they understand each other's business strengths and weaknesses and can fill in the gaps? The doctor told me she gives huge credit for her business success to her manager, whom she views as a vital partner. Ross Perot said "You can buy my business out from under me, but leave me my key people and in five years we'll be back better than ever!" Trying to explain to the class the fundamental importance of the team approach, a truck driver in one of my seminars blurted out "One [truck company] owner can't drive thirty trucks by himself!" And I add, nor can one doctor.

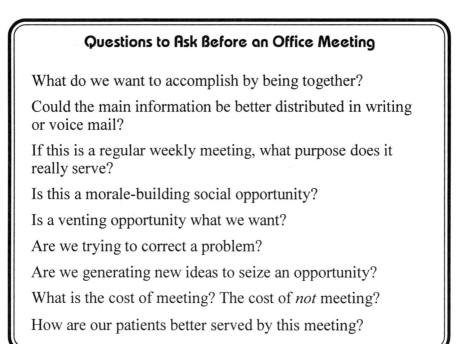

Questions to Ask Before an Office Meeting

What do we want to accomplish by being together?

Could the main information be better distributed in writing or voice mail?

If this is a regular weekly meeting, what purpose does it really serve?

Is this a morale-building social opportunity?

Is a venting opportunity what we want?

Are we trying to correct a problem?

Are we generating new ideas to seize an opportunity?

What is the cost of meeting? The cost of *not* meeting?

How are our patients better served by this meeting?

Different Types of Meetings

You don't use the same size pot to prepare every meal. You don't use the same meeting format to satisfy all of your needs. Try different types of meetings for a broader range of results.

Morning Huddle. Try a daily 10 to 15 minute stand-up meeting to frame the day before seeing your first patient. Topics: What opportunities do you see in our schedule? Where do we have hurdles to overcome today? What needs to be said now, so that each of us can be focused 100% on patient care today?

End of Day Debriefing. Quick up-and-down recap of what worked today and what didn't. Where do we need to focus for improvement — systems, communication, equipment, training, etc.? What issues need to be addressed so that each person can leave work behind and focus on families and friends?

Weekly One-Hour Staff Meeting. Opportunity for more in-depth analysis of where this team soars and where it lays an egg. How can we improve the patient flow? What are the patients saying about us? Who deserves a pat on the back? Who dealt successfully with the biggest challenge? Who's the hero of the week? Michael Egan, D.D.S., a general dentist in Hartford, Connecticut, with a full time staff of five, relates that their weekly staff meetings absolutely energize and focus the team.

Lunch and Learn. Once a month, meet informally during lunch; have one team member conduct a 20-minute training session that's followed by lots of discussion on applying this information to the office. Christian Loetscher, D.D.S., M.S., an oral and maxillofacial surgeon in Norcross, Georgia, has found periodic meetings to discuss office procedures allow the business office and clinical staff to gain understanding of each person's role.

Quarterly meeting. Excellent occasion to review progress toward your goals. Are we on track to make year-end predictions? Would it be appropriate to stretch our goals at this time? Discuss where adjustments can be made. Gain commitment to a five-week experiment to try a new procedure. In-service training is also a valuable part of quarterly staff meetings.

Annual meeting. Review the year past and the year ahead. Measure progress. Raise the bar higher to make the new one the best year yet.

Office picnic and holiday party. (Yes, these are meetings, sort of!) Acknowledge the *total team* by including families; games, contests, and skits interweave lives. Acknowledge contributions made by spouses, parents, and children. Present awards for accomplishments.

Ground Rules for Meetings that Work

Legendary Green Bay Packers coach, Vince Lombardi, believed success is attainable when we master the basics. He started one post-game debriefing with, "This is a football." Has your team mastered the basics for productive meetings? Here are some suggested ground rules for conduct in your meetings.

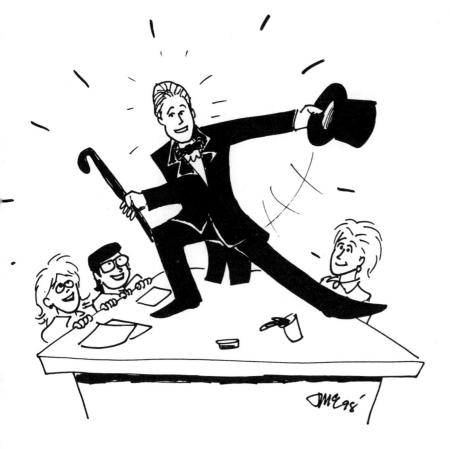

MEETINGS STIMULATE CREATIVITY!

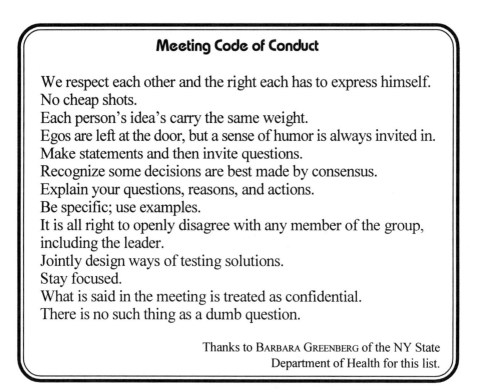

Meeting Code of Conduct

We respect each other and the right each has to express himself.
No cheap shots.
Each person's idea's carry the same weight.
Egos are left at the door, but a sense of humor is always invited in.
Make statements and then invite questions.
Recognize some decisions are best made by consensus.
Explain your questions, reasons, and actions.
Be specific; use examples.
It is all right to openly disagree with any member of the group,
including the leader.
Jointly design ways of testing solutions.
Stay focused.
What is said in the meeting is treated as confidential.
There is no such thing as a dumb question.

Thanks to BARBARA GREENBERG of the NY State
Department of Health for this list.

And for meetings that bond:

1. Have a beginning time and stick to it. Being flexible for
latecomers backfires: the on-time people are penalized and a subtle
signal is sent that deadlines are only suggestions.

*2. Schedule the best part of the meeting as the first agenda
item.* On-time attendance at my weekly meeting shot up when
I moved the fun "heroes of the week" part of the meeting from the
end to the beginning.

3. Use an agenda. Time is money; demonstrate your good
stewardship of the organization's resources by not winging it.

*4. Circulate agenda-related items at least one day prior to the
meeting.* When attendees can read the handouts and do their homework
before the meeting, the discussion has added depth.

5. Brief people before meetings. Key decisions deserve more
thought than just a gut reaction following a few minutes of discussion.

6. Appoint people to be in charge of different agenda items. Face it. Always having the same leader is predictable, mind numbing, and innovation killing. Mixing it up will give added depth of discussion, higher interest, and as Einstein observed, "it takes more than one brain for real breakthrough thinking."

7. A brief education segment is appropriate. It's a fast-changing world. Your team has probably gone through radical change in the last couple of years. Keep the group mind moving forward at the same pace.

8. Set an example by being prepared. Looking casual is reassuring; being casual is not.

9. Compute meeting costs. Your practice is investing approximately $15 to $50 per hour per person to hold staff meetings. Ask yourself, "How can we maximize our productivity during this meeting and create added value for our patients?"

10. Could you write a detailed memo instead of having a meeting? If you frequently spend time discussing office procedures, perhaps the cause is a communication issue and can be handled better in writing or by smaller, focused meetings.

11. Have someone record meeting decisions and distribute within 24 to 48 hours after the meeting. If it is important enough for a meeting, then it is important enough to be recorded and followed up.

12. End on time. Peak performance teams start on time and end on time. Have someone act as an "FTA" (forward the action) person. Every agenda item should have an estimated timeline that is adhered to. If the business at hand cannot be accomplished within the time frame requested, ask permission for more time or place it at the top of unfinished business for the next meeting.

13. Keep good ideas alive by appreciating that not everyone accepts change in the same way. When it comes to change, people fall into three categories: 20% enjoy change. (Gayle: "That's a great idea! We should have been doing it that way all along."); 50% are willing to change but cautious, (Kevin: "I like your idea, but I don't know. Send me something in writing, I'll study it."); and 30% are so uncomfortable with change they put their energies into slowing it down, stopping it, or trying to go back to the way it used to be (Kathy: "It'll never work. We tried that already. You won't get approval. It costs too much. At my last job we did it the right way.") At meetings where tough issues are being discussed, look closely and you will see the strata of all three layers. Here is one reason good ideas die in meetings: on the *first hearing* of a new idea the opposition will be approximately 80% of the people in attendance. Suggestion: don't take it personally. Don't even see it as rejection. In fact, a pretty good strategy is to smile deep inside, understand that the universe is still working properly, and persevere.

Meetings are a FUNdamental™ element of peak performance teams. They should be **focused** on moving toward your vision and maintaining open lines of communication. Everyone should have an **understanding** of the agenda items and come fully prepared to participate, so that the cycle of **never-ending improvement** is perpetuated. The average dental team views meetings as "lost production time." Peak performance teams understand that this is truly the most highly productive time of their week!

Doug Smart

Doug is a speaker, consultant, and radio personality. He is the author of TimeSmart: How Real People Get Things Done at Work, TimeSmart: How Real People Really Get Things Done at Home and Reach for the Stars. As president of Doug Smart Seminars, he conducts programs tailored to helping business professionals in healthcare, education, sales, industry, and government increase personal productivity and organizational ability — while reducing stress! Using ideas gained in working with over 900 groups in six years, his insight is unique and up to the minute. He has spoken for organizations as diverse as Tulane University Medical Center, LSU Medical Center, National Institutes of Health, City of Hope Hospital, University of Illinois, and Vistacon.

Doug keeps current with membership in the American Society for Training and Development, National Speakers Association, Georgia Speakers Association, and Meeting Professionals International.

For information on scheduling a seminar or keynote, you can contact Doug at Doug Smart Seminars. Phone (770) 587-9784, Fax (770) 587-1050, E-mail: DougSmart.Seminars@worldnet.att.net.

Words of Wisdom

Having meetings which center on discussing the importance of our daily routines creates a sense of belonging and accomplishment... a clear understanding that what each person does has relevance and is important to the success of the organization is an essential element of any team.

DR. ALAN HINKLE
McLean, VA

We have daily clearing and debriefing meetings in which we make sure everyone is doing well and if they are not, we see how we can support them. These meetings also allow us to do daily planning as a team and acknowledge one another.

DR. STEVE KAIL
Alamo, TN

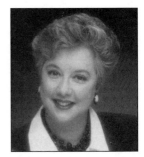

Chapter Nine

'Patterns, Impressions' & Your Leadership Potential: Break Through Tools for Effective Leadership

Linda Drevenstedt, RDH, M.S.

"To move the world, we must first move ourselves." — SOCRATES

Since the mid 1970's practice management information for dentists, including seminars, books, training, and coaching has reproduced like rabbits. Yet with all of these aids, dentists still struggle, bouncing from one source to another, searching for sure-fire ways to a more profitable and fulfilling practice. Dentists want high performance teams, "raving fan" patients who refer more patients, and the lifestyle of successful professionals. Why don't these thousands of dental professionals have what they desire? The answer lies in their leadership abilities.

As a new millennium approaches, dental businesses require leadership in ways never demanded before. Changes in reimbursement, technology, social trends, and a myriad of other changes are forcing dentists to develop new skills. The most important skill is leadership — the ability to guide people and a business to the vision of the leader. This definition implies that a leader is someone who knows where he or she is going. The Bible tells us that without a vision people perish; the leader, as well as the followers. Your vision is a clear picture of where you as the leader want your practice to be in the future. Leadership starts with leading yourself. If you have no vision for your future, or an incomplete vision, guiding your staff and your business into an effective future will indeed be difficult.

This chapter guides you through processes and actions to assist in clarifying your future. The clearer your vision, the easier it is to have that future become reality. Nevertheless, the creation of *your* vision is not easy. The work will be ongoing. The vision changes and expands the more your leadership potential grows. But at each growth level there are coaches, mentors, and advisors available to assist you. Never rest on your laurels. Resting does not lift your spirit and certainly does not inspire your staff or patients.

Your current practice is a consequence of your past self-concept, beliefs, and paradigms. It evolved as a direct result of your vision. You enlarge your vision by enlarging your beliefs and paradigms while growing as a person and as a leader. As you grow, you become a more effective leader, helping the staff members who choose to follow you to grow. As the people you lead grows, your business grows.

Because your vision will change as you grow in the awareness of options, your vision must be revisited annually. Let's start your journey.

Leadership Tools

Leadership begins and ends with you. As the leader of a dental practice, you are the one who gives the team direction. Your moods, personal life, goals (or lack of goals), drive, boredom, commitment (or lack of commitment) to growth and progress, and your values all effect your practice.

To clarify your vision, make a personal inventory of where you are now. Take out a sheet of paper and title the sheet "My Practice." Draw a line down the center of the paper. On the right side write where you are now; on the left side write where you would like to be. Getting things on paper is the most important step in any of the processes in this chapter. Once you have the pages completed, you have the rough draft of your personal vision for the future.

Next is gap analysis. Identify the gap between where you are now and where you want to be. To get where you want to be involves *change*. Get used to that word, for it is the only way you will grow as a leader and be able to face the rapidly changing future of dentistry. Learning to move yourself into change is essential. Making progress either personally or professionally will *always* require change. Your ability to become an expert "change agent" for yourself, your practice, your staff, and your patients is vital to your leadership tool kit.

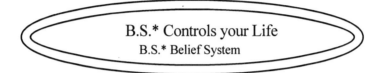

B.S.* Controls your Life
B.S.* Belief System

Why is change so difficult for most people? It is based on B.S.* (*Belief System*) Your brain creates your reality. Your brain is full of information that has been stored for your whole lifetime. Much of the data has been stored without censor, without review, without judgment, and without your knowledge. Only a percentage of your life is controlled by your conscious mind. Your subconscious mind influences most of your thoughts and actions. The subconscious mind is the repository of all of your impressions, opinions, feelings, and experiences. It is all there. Information you received as a child, as a student, as a scout, as a boy or as a girl. A Talmudic teaching sums this up, "We don't see things as they are. We see things as we are."

Many of your actions evolve from your subconscious impressions. This process often has no judgment about the value of the impression; the impression is merely stored. Just as a copy machine does not evaluate the value of what you copy, your mind, particularly when you are young, does not evaluate the data stored in your subconscious. As you grow into adolescence and adulthood, impressions create who you are and how you act. Your beliefs then filter what goes into your mind. Those things which fit your beliefs go in and those which don't are filtered out by your current beliefs. Do you remember the song from South Pacific "You've Got to Be Carefully Taught"? You are taught by those who impress you: parents, bosses, professors, role models (positive and negative), church or synagogue leaders, relatives, siblings, friends, acquaintances, anyone or anything that you have interaction with. Your growth as a leader will force you to tap into the subconscious part of your mind and begin to change those impressions that no longer serve you.

As a leader you have a Belief System about Leadership and Leaders. What follows is a Leadership Tool which helps address your leadership beliefs.

On a sheet of paper answer the following questions:
1. Who are the people who have been your role model leaders?
2. What are the attributes and qualities of leadership of these people?
3. Which of these qualities in your opinion is positive? (Put a "+" by it.)
4. Which of these attributes is in your opinion negative? (Put a "—" by it.)

The items marked negative are often a part of your own leadership profile. Negative experiences, particularly with role models, can strongly, yet randomly, influence your belief system. Those may include examples such as these:

Pressure to perform at school, possibly with little praise.
Strict rules to follow to gain approval.
Push to perform perfectly while being told you did not measure up.

These experiences can often translate into leadership Belief Systems that might suggest the following: necessity to perform perfectly, necessity to be strict and control others, verbally or silently, anger at self and others for not meeting high expectations, fear of disapproval from others, or worry over not making everyone happy.

How do you break free of your Belief System? You choose to change your mind. If you are happy and content in all areas of you life, please skip to the next chapter now. If you are dissatisfied with the way things are, read on. Your precursor for change is the dissatisfaction with the way things are.

The primary thing that has prevented change before now is your Belief System and your pride in that Belief System. Pride protects the ego from that uncomfortable thought: "I've been wrong about _____." What is really wrong is the belief that someone or something other than *you* has to change for things on your list to change. Change starts with you. Taking 100% responsibility for where you are now is the first step.

Barriers to Effective Leadership

The three primary barriers of ineffective leadership paradigms are anger, fear, and worry. The journey to conquer, control, reduce, reframe, and eliminate the barriers to your success takes persistence, but builds character. Ben Franklin gives us the best advice, "resolve to perform that which you ought. Perform without fail that which you resolve." *Keep on keeping on* is the modern twist on Ben Franklin's quote. Work with the exercises provided to break through these barriers. Once you can lead yourself, you can lead your practice and others into the greater realization of potential.

Mishandled anger is destructive and our first barrier. Ineffective responses to anger usually involve suppression or inappropriate expression of anger. A leader who suppresses this powerful emotion often misdirects the anger, becoming a victim of, as Zig Ziglar calls it, "Kick the Cat Syndrome" — releasing anger on the wrong person. On the other hand is the dentist with the short fuse who throws instruments, yells, or in some other way alienates staff and patients alike. People with high self esteem (the ones you want as team members) will not stay in a rage filled environment.

The second barrier to effective leadership is fear. Fear is a highly personal experience, varying from one individual to the next. Innate natural fears, such as fear of falling, are there to protect you from harm. Your body responds with a sympathetic nervous system response. Your brain is programmed to avoid danger to your body. Think of a time when you were driving and someone suddenly pulled out in front of you. Your body sent a shot of adrenaline to help you respond quickly and you slammed on your brakes. Once the incident was over, and a brief moment of racing heart and held breath, you took a deep breath and returned to the drive. Here, the adrenaline caused a positive and productive response.

In daily life there are few life-threatening dangers, yet there are many fears. Stress is a form of fear in daily life: stress over bills, employees, children, and a myriad of other life situations. Fear in the form of stress keeps our bodies in a constant state of "fight or flight." With stress, however, adrenaline rushes in and uses the body's energy in non-productive ways. The quickened heart rate and additional hormonal response causes us to become impatient, short tempered, and intolerant of others; this leads to strained relationships, unfulfilled expectations, and lack of respect.

Feeling powerless, you look for something to ease or block the stress or fear. Thus, the negative habits lead to irrational attempts at controlling or rescuing others or an inability to act. As a leader, fear can keep you from addressing your staff's poor performance, taking your practice to another level, or having your vision accomplished.

The third barrier to effective leadership is worry — which is simply negative visioning. Worry creates negative impulses in your subconscious, saps your energy, and keeps you either future focused (i.e., worrying about what will happen), or past focused (i.e., worrying about what happened). Worry builds walls that keep you isolated from honest communication with others. When you worry over a staff member's quitting if you don't give her the raise she wants, you may not communicate honestly with her. While you are in a worry mode, you cannot be 100% aware of others, or hear what they are saying to you. For example, if you are worried about having enough money for payroll, you cannot really hear the concerns of new patients in your practice.

The following leadership tools will help you reframe your beliefs about anger, fear and worry. By working through each of these exercises, you will gain strength as a leader.

Resolving Anger

The following is an effective tool to handle anger. The next time one of your staff angers you, do the following:

1. Give yourself permission to feel angry. Anger is a signal that something needs to be handled. Often a boundary has not been set or communicated; a need has not been identified; or an expectation has not clearly been explained.

2. Take time to think about your anger and to choose an appropriate time to discuss the situation with the person. Find a private place with no time pressure to discuss your anger with the person.

3. Be willing to reframe your opinion of the situation or event. Be willing to suspend judgment of the person.

4. State your anger clearly:

I am angry because _____

This makes me angry because (<u>state results of actions or behaviors of the other person</u>.)

5. Ask how the two of you can resolve the problem. State what you want to have happen. Ask her to state what she wants to have happen and tell you what she needs to meet your expectation.

6. Be willing to release your need to have it "only your way," or the need to be "right." Is the expectation you have realistic? (Expecting <u>never</u> to have a cancellation is not realistic.) Listen to the other person. Steven Covey says "Seek first to understand, then to be understood." Does this staff member need training, materials, or a new system to meet the expectation?

7. Make requests and set boundaries. Clearly state expectations and boundaries. Others are not responsible for "mind reading."

8. Realize that setting boundaries and stating expectations can cause frustration for other people. You are responsible for taking care of yourself and your practice, and for setting the standards for your practice. The staff member may not have the temperament or behaviors you need for the job you are expecting her/him to do.

9. Clearly define an action plan to resolve the situation.

Remember you have a choice. You can hold on to your old way of dealing with anger or you can heal and grow by breaking down this barrier. Use your personal resolve to continue to handle your anger in these new ways.

Fear Worksheet

Make a list of the things you fear. The list should also include specific fears about your practice, your staff, your family, your health, your income, and your future.

Examples: Failing at something, not doing something right; having your feelings hurt; debt; being wrong; change; rejection; "what others think"; disappointing parents, spouse, or children; not being perfect enough; etc.

Consider what your fear is costing you and what you might gain by changing your current fear/stress pattern? Breaking through the fear barrier requires risk and the willingness to stretch your comfort zone. (Stretching your comfort zone is a constant part of leadership growth.)

Go back to your list of fears and begin to "walk" into each one with a changed perception. What follows is a fear-busting tool which will allow you to reframe your Belief System fears.

Fear Busting Tool

Write out a positive statement that would dispel the fear. This becomes a positive affirmation that reprograms your belief system. Read it out loud and with enthusiasm several times every day, each time with more intensity and congruency.

Example:

Fear: I am afraid I will not have enough patients to keep my practice growing.

Affirmation: My patients appreciate quality dentistry and happily make referrals.

Take action to resolve the fear. Action cures fear and stretches your comfort zone.

Example: Learn to build a referral based practice from others that have success in this area. Enroll in a communications course to increase case acceptance.

Worry Worksheet

1. List the people, places, and things that are on your current worry list.

2. List why you are worried about each person, place, or thing.

3. Determine how each worry affects you.

4. Imagine the absolute worst thing that could happen if your worry came true. How would you handle that worst outcome?

5. Take what actions you can today to prevent the negative outcome.

6. Imagine the best outcome. What actions would you take to prepare for success?

If there is no action you can take, then turn it over to a higher power, and **let it go**! It is not yours to solve, fix, or change. Norman Vincent Peale in the <u>Power of Positive Thinking</u> says, "Faith is the one power against which worry cannot stand."

Once you have controlled anger, fear, and worry (the three barriers to great leadership) you will be more relaxed, your relationships with staff will be improved, and you can better lead your team. People are their happiest when they are embraced by achievement and accomplishment.

Linda Drevenstedt, RDH, M.S.

Linda Drevenstedt, RDH, M.S. is President of The Drevenstedt Group, Inc. She and her team of professionals assist dental practices in running better dental businesses. She has been a practice management consultant for over ten years. An expert in her field, she has been published and quoted in numerous state and national professional journals and she lectures at major conferences.

Ms. Drevenstedt's diverse experience includes: dental assisting, dental hygiene, and managing a multi-specialty group practice with a staff of 45. She holds undergraduate degrees in Dental Hygiene and Business Management, and a Masters Degree in Health Care Administration. In addition, she is a member of the National Speaker's Association, the American Society for Training and Development and the Academy of Dental Management Consultants.

She can be contacted at (800) 242-7648 or E-mail: drevgrp@aol.com

Words of Wisdom

Sharing the same vision is important in order to achieve goals and (it is) rewarding when those goals are met.

DR. DEBRA KING
Atlanta, GA

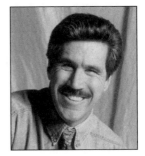

Chapter Ten

'Cementing' Relationships with Specialists:
Team Approach to Case Acceptance

Paul Homoly, D.D.S.

*"Many people know how to work hard; many others know how
to play well; but the rarest talent in the world is the ability
to introduce elements of playfulness into work, and to put some
constructive labor into our leisure."* — SIDNEY J. HARRIS

The advances in dental technology and therapeutics have changed
the way general dentists and specialists work together. As these new
fields continue to grow, so must the referral systems between offices.
Cosmetic and implant dentistry is creating greater demands on the
relationship between the offices of the general practitioner and
specialist. The simple, uncomplicated referral for specialty procedures
is giving way to more interactive and interdisciplinary relationships.

The advances in dental technology and therapeutics have changed
the way general dentist and specialists work together. And, as these new
fields continue to grow, so must the referral system between offices.
The traditional referral relationship worked fine for third molar
removal, periodontal surgery, or orthodontic care; however, such
minimal interoffice treatment planning and patient management do not

suffice for complex cosmetic and implant referrals. Here, an informed and well-coordinated team approach to dental care is essential. Treatment plans, budget and insurance considerations, and diagnostic information must be fully shared with patient and specialist.

Just before a seminar, I was approached by three periodontists. One cornered me whining, "I'll tell you what's wrong with most general dentists I work with, they're shot blockers. They unsell more dentistry than they sell. I'd starve if I had to rely on their referrals. They need to get their acts together."

"Amen," cheered his buddies. "How do we get them to change?"

Later that same day, a general dentist handed me a radiograph. It showed seven implants — two were failing and one was unrestorable. "I sent my patient to an oral surgeon for an implant evaluation. Nine months later the patient returned with a mouth full of implants and couldn't afford the restorative dentistry. What can I do to keep that from happening again?"

Like the disgruntled couple who confess each other's sins but fail to see their own, dental team members often point accusing fingers without recognizing their own contribution to the problem.

The Honeymoon is Over

Here, on the other hand, is a team approach situation. A new patient comes into the general dentist's office. After examining the patient, the dentist concludes the best way to replace the missing posterior teeth is with dental implants and recommends seeing an oral surgeon for evaluation.

If the general dentist is lucky, the patient will take his advice and seek the opinion of the specialist. Following his examination, the specialist describes the use of dental implants and shows the patient visual aids and gives her a consent form to read at home. Just as the specialist is ready to escort her to the door, the patient asks the knockout question, "How much will my insurance pay for this work?"

The specialist winces, "Didn't your general dentist explain all this to you?"

"No, the only thing he did was send me here and I'm not sure I can afford all this. How much does a reline cost?"

As illustrated, patients are more likely to become disoriented and reluctant when the general and specialty dental teams are not in harmony. The communication problems which create such "disharmony," and patient confusions are remedied by an organized sharing of technical, financial, and patient information and responsibilities.

To Have and To Hold

There's an important distinction between teamwork and team harmony. Teamwork is the technical aspect — copying records, duplicating radiographs, referral letters, follow-up care, telephone calls, and so on. Teamwork, in short, is behind-the-scenes work. Team harmony is the relationship aspect of the team — cheerful attitudes, amiable communication, collegiality. Team harmony is what the patient sees and experiences and hence, has the greatest impact on treatment acceptance. The optimal team approach is a blend of teamwork and team harmony.

Team Approach Courtship

Let's revisit the scenario when the new patient enters the general dentist's office, this time looking at the courtship sequence to case acceptance. With a team approach the general dentist is:

- Building a solid relationship with the patient.
- Determining whether the patient is interested in minor dental care or comprehensive care involving specialty procedures.
- Determining the patient's annual budget for dental care.
- Comprehensive examination and treatment planning.
- Recommending and informing regarding specialty procedures.
- Communicating the plan and recommending that portion of the plan that falls within the patient's budget.

Building Solid Relationships

You must first determine whether the patient is interested in treating his chief complaint only (minor tooth repair) or in a lifetime strategy for dental health. The traditional approach to care occurs when a general dentist spots something that is out of his/her technical training and refers the patient to the specialist. Wrong! The role of the general dentist in the team approach is to act as the anchor office. Patients rely on their general dentists for help and support in making decisions regarding the recommendations of specialists; and so the foundation of the team to patient care is the patient's relationship with the general dentist's office.

Those patients interested in treating only their chief dental complaint should receive that care. If, however, once the chief complaint is relieved, the patient still has significant dental breakdown, you should repeat your offer of providing a strategy for lifetime dental health. Continue to explore options until you can fully determine the patient's needs and interest level. Once their initial concerns have been met, place them in the recall system for follow-up care.

If the patient opts for a comprehensive lifetime approach to dental health, the general dentist's office performs a complete examination, collects all diagnostic tools (mounted study models, photographs, etc.), and develops a complete treatment plan. Understanding the specialist's fees and treatment criteria, the general dentist can estimate fees and duration of treatment, allowing the patient to make sound decisions.

Determining the Patient's Annual Budget for Dental Care

A large part of building lasting relationships with patients is determining their annual spending plan for dental care. Since most patients have never given thought to incorporating this type of spending into their personal budgets, assisting them in this financial aspect of care is one of the dental teams most complex challenges. This topic is discussed in detail in <u>Dentists: Endangered Species—A Survival Guide for Fee-For-Service Care</u>. For a few guidelines on conducting this conversation, consider the following:

During the initial appointment, say "I'm good at staying within a budget, if I know I need to. Have you thought about your budget for dental care?" and, at the following appointment, "Last appointment, I mentioned it was important to me to stay within your budget. Give me an idea what would be a comfortable budget for you and I'll make sure we stay within it."

Please note that the team approach to care includes your financial coordinator in all conversations concerning patient payment. Once you have a ballpark figure to organize your treatment plan, allow your business office to assist the patient with the details. Your role on the team is to responsibly diagnose, communicate, and treat dental health concerns.

Time for Referral

The time is right to refer a patient for specialty care when the patient:

- Cannot continue planned treatment without specialized care.
- Is aware of the estimated fees and duration of treatment for specialty care.
- Has a solid relationship with the general dentist and staff.

The dialogue surrounding the referral process is key. Let's eavesdrop on a conversation between a patient and general dentist who is about to refer to a specialist for placement of implants. They are seated in the consultation area, the patient's chart closed in front of him, a telephone on a side table nearby;

"Mrs. McBucks, do you remember when I told you some of your treatment would be completed by a specialist?" asks Dr. DuRight.

"Yes I do, Dr. DuRight. You said that I needed dental implants and someone else would do that work."

"Let me tell you about the specialist who will be seeing you. Her name is Dr. Kristen Homoly. She's a gum and bone specialist and her office is just one block from here. We'll give you a map, but it's easy to find. Dr. Homoly is one of the finest specialists in the area. I've been working with her for five years, and our patients really enjoy her. She has advanced training in implant dentistry and patients come from all over the region to see her. Do you have questions or comments about why you're seeing her?" asks the general dentist.

"Will I have the implants done on the first visit?"

"No. Dr. Homoly will examine you first, probably take a few x-rays, and then outline a plan of care for you. She'll communicate the plan to me also, so I'll know where you are in treatment every step of the way."

"The total fees for your implants have already been estimated within the treatment plan that I have done for you. I estimate Dr. Homoly's fees to be in the $6,000 range. You'll pay those fees directly to her office, which will handle all of the insurance claims related to your care with them. She has already seen your x-rays, and we've talked about your case."

"Yes, I remember you telling me this. Plus, you mentioned it in a letter I received from your office. When should I go and see Dr. Homoly?"

"Let's call her now. Ginger is her receptionist. I'm sure that we can make arrangements for you."

"This is Dr. DuRight calling and I'm referring Mrs. McBucks to Dr. Homoly for implant placement. Is Dr. Homoly available to come to the telephone?"

"Dr. Homoly is with a patient right now, but I'll be glad to have her return your call. May I give your patient appointment and referral information?" asks Ginger.

"Let me ask her," replies the general dentist. "Mrs. McBucks, I have Ginger, Dr. Homoly's receptionist, on the line; for your convenience, she's available to schedule your appointment right now. Would you like to talk with her?"

Dr. DuRight hands the telephone to the patient, who discusses appointment procedures while he makes the referral entry in her record.

Following the conversation, Mrs. McBucks is brought to the front desk and receives referral information — maps and introductory letters.

"You'll love Dr. Homoly," says Lily, the scheduling coordinator. "All our patients say the nicest things about her, and her staff. Ginger is the scheduling coordinator for their practice. She and I attend a lot of continuing education together. You'll like her. I'll make sure they have the x-rays and models needed to plan your case."

"Thank you so much. You've made this easy for me," smiles Mrs. McBucks as she leaves.

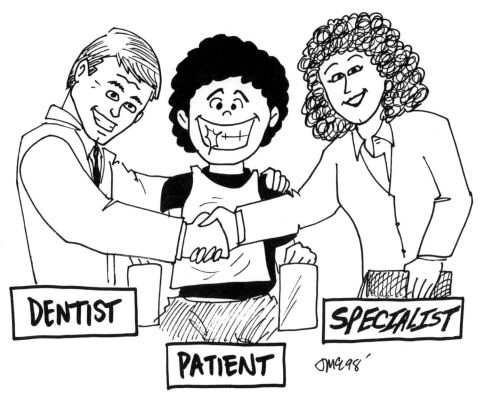

HARMONY BETWEEN REFERRING PRACTICES IS ESSENTIAL!

Great Referrals

Let's analyze this dialogue and discover the components of great referrals.

- The referral was not a surprise.
- The patient was informed of the possibility early in the relationship.
- Strong testimony for the credibility of the specialist's team was given.
- Enthusiasm about the referral and the patient taking the next step in treatment was demonstrated.
- Remove unknowns from the referral process. Let patient know what to expect.
- Give the patient the sense of your continued involvement with her care.
- Remind the patient of the expected fees and duration of treatment.
- Personally make the referring telephone call with the patient present.
- Encourage the patient to make the initial appointment while still in your office.
- Provide maps, telephone number, and brochures describing the specialty procedure.
- Staff offers strong endorsement of the specialty team.
- Follow-up by communicating your intended treatment plan, estimated fees, and time frame with the specialist. Also, forward all pertinent x-rays and study models.

Can you recall the distinction between team work and team harmony? How many aspect of a great referral relate to team harmony — attitude, good communication, collegiality? Great referrals are 90% team harmony and 10% team work.

In the Specialist's Office

During the patient's first appointment with the specialist, it should be obvious to the patient that:

★   The specialty team is aware of the patient's treatment plan
★   The offices respect each other and enjoy working together
★   All diagnostic materials have been forwarded to the specialty team
★   Insurance and financial information has been forwarded

Here's a sample dialogue accomplishing these criteria in the first few minutes of the patient's experience.

"Mrs. McBucks, welcome to our office. I'm Ginger. We spoke on the telephone a few days ago. Lily, from Dr. DuRight's, office has forwarded your x-rays, models, and medical history and insurance information to our office. Would you please double check this information and sign here to indicate that my information is correct? Dr. Homoly is excited about your visit with us today and is prepared to see you momentarily."

"Good morning, Mrs. McBucks, I'm Dr. Homoly. It's a pleasure meeting another one of Dr. DuRight's patients. I've discussed your care with him and I'm well aware of your treatment plan. You made a great decision when you chose Dr. DuRight as your dentist. He and I have treated patients together for years, and I'm impressed with his thoroughness and skill. We've received your x-rays and study models, and today I will examine you and we'll talk about how we can best help you."

If the patient refuses specialty procedures, it's a direct result of poor preparation prior to the specialist's case presentation. Case acceptance is predictable when each office fulfills its role. When patients feel the center of attention in each office, and feel appreciated and important, saying 'yes' to treatment is easy. Unlike battling married couples and their weary children, team treatment offices and their patients can learn to grow and harmonize together, never regretting saying "I do."

Team Harmony Quotient

In regard to your relationship with referring practices, place a check mark by those items that are currently implemented in your practice.

General Dentistry Teams

- Build strong relationship with patient prior to referral.
- The entire team offers testimony and endorsement of specialty team.
- Congratulates patient on a wise decision.
- Pre-frame first visit with specialist. Let patients know what to expect.
- Inform patient that you will continue to monitor progress.
- Remind patient of estimated fees for specialty procedures.
- Place referral call in the presence of the patient.
- Make initial appointment while patient is still in your office.
- Provide maps, telephone numbers, and brochures on specialty procedure.
- Sends complete patient information and records to specialty office.
- Continue contact with specialist throughout treatment sequence.

Specialty Dental Teams

- Welcome patient to practice.
- Confirm receipt of personal, financial, medical and diagnostic information.
- Reinforce patient's decision to continue with comprehensive care.
- Praise referring dentist and team. Emphasize strong working relationship.
- Show confidence in general dentist's diagnostic and clinical skills.
- Complete examination. Confirm general dentist's assessment or convey to the patient alternative options.
- Communicate directly with general dentist on patient's needs. Do not send messages through patient.
- Have an understanding of general dentist's financial policies and patient's expectations.
- Continue communication throughout treatment sequence.

Dr. Paul Homoly

Dr. Homoly presents his work internationally, is active on the national teaching level, and designs business and marketing plans for general dentists and specialists. He practiced restorative dentistry in Charlotte, NC for 20 years, and is one of the rare practitioners who excels in both the clinical and managerial aspects of dentistry.

Paul is one of the top-rated speakers and trainers in dentistry. He offers a one-day program based on his book <u>Dentists: An Endangered Species</u>. Additionally, Dr. Homoly conducts workshops on marketing, personal and practice development, and case presentation skills. For more information on how Dr. Paul Homoly can serve your organization call (800) 294-9370, Fax (704) 522-9961, or E-mail: <u>phomoly@aol.com</u>

Free by fax: Want a letter designed to go to patients that explains why minimizing dental insurance and avoiding managed care is good for them? Just fax your letterhead with your name and fax number with the words "Minimizing Insurance" to (704) 522-9961.

Words of Wisdom

Team is promoted by focusing on the patient, not on the individual team member. If our goal is to welcome the patient on time and to perform excellent dentistry and collect our fees, we all must work for the patient so that we can succeed as a group and share in the success with decent compensation and bonus when we excel.

DR. PATRICIA HUDETZ
Naperville, IL

Our team offers their time and talent to our community with a day of free dentistry. Everyone rallies around the cause... Excitement is in the air because we are ALL involved in making a difference for others.

DR. CLAYTON CUMMINGS
Nashville, TN

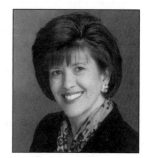

Chapter Eleven

'Brushing' Up on Coaching Skills: Effective Coaching Techniques

Vicki McManus, RDH

"One of the best ways to persuade others is with your ears — by listening to them." — DEAN RUSK

For many years we have thought of management consultants as experts that come into our practices and "fix" them or in some way "do things to our practice." What we are now seeing is an emergence of partnering with clients, more of a coaching relationship, rather than a consultative one.

Before you enter into a coaching relationship there are several questions that you should ask yourself. Am I coachable? Am I willing to make changes? Meaning, are you willing to listen and follow the guidance of your coach. This does not mean that you are a passive participant blindly following their lead. It simply means that you maintain open dialogue and communication with your coach.

Now that we have a dedicated team, how do we sustain peak performance? Effective coaching achieves effective results!

By definition, anyone can be a coach. In fact, we all engage in coaching on some level. Whenever you initiate a conversation to affect a specific result, you are coaching. The most effective coaching conversation has a clearly defined purpose and a limited element of chance. This coaching requires training, an ongoing view toward the end results, and methodological skill.

Following the <u>ASTD Trainer's Manual: Coaching</u>, let's put a working definition of coaching in place. First of all, effective coaching is built by effective conversation, and effective coaching conversations are built on three key elements.

1. Creates C.A.N.I.!® — Constant And Never-ending Improvement
2. Results oriented
3. Disciplined

To put it all together, Effective Coaching involves a disciplined conversation between a leader and an individual or a team that results in constant and never-ending improvement.

Effective Coaching that results in C.A.N.I.!® begins with the coach's values. It is *not* about using a few behavioral tricks or clever communication ploys to manipulate others. Rather, it is about sharing beliefs in human competency, peak performance, and the value of coaching.

Let's look at some common beliefs of outstanding coaches. Coaches believe people want to be competent. Given the opportunity and appropriate support, they will strive to become more competent. They know their staff must be given opportunity to demonstrate their competency on a continual basis.

Committed coaches believe that control-based management is not good practice nor conducive to long-term growth or improved performances. Positive results are achieved and sustained by total team commitment to top performance. Coaches both reinforce and model this commitment and its results. In addition, effective coaches never stop working to enhance the self-esteem and confidence of each team member. This is accomplished by by clearly defining their roles, investing in ongoing training, creating challenges, allowing for learning experiences through correcting mistakes, and rewarding hard work. Penny Reed will discuss this aspect of coaching in greater detail in her chapter on 'rewarding and motivating your team.'

There are five essential characteristics of effective coaching: conversation-balance, measurability, shared responsibility, context, and respect.

The first characteristic is balance. Coaching conversations are not one-sided; they require give and take. Open and flexible, these conversations question and share with everyone's full participation. In some conversations, the coach will be the initiator and facilitator; in others, the reverse.

The second characteristic is measurability. Each conversation focuses on what can be improved. The coach is direct and specific and encourages others to be also. Inherent in these conversations is the mutual understanding of the expectations and behaviors necessary for the desired performance improvements. Thus acknowledging these expectations, each member of the team is measured against them.

The third characteristic is shared responsibility. Dentists who act as coaches for their teams understand that their success is dependent on the work ethic, attitude, and performance of every member of the team. There are no "management vs. employee" situations. Everyone is responsible for creating an environment of constant and never-ending improvement, and every conversation must reflect this level of shared responsibility.

The fourth characteristic of superior coaching conversations is context. The form of the conversation should be distinct and easily reproduced, while the context changes and expands according to the goal of the conversation. Creating the shape and flow of coaching conversations is a learned skill and must be practiced on a daily basis. One of the primary functions of a coach and consultant for dental teams is coaching creation of the context of their conversations. By refining their language skills, they can support the flow of the conversation to produce measurable results.

The final characteristic of coaching conversations is respect. The leader must communicate respect for the people being coached. Rather than dominating the conversation, the coach actually solicits comments. The result of effective coaching is that the persons being coached participate in the solution to the challenge and 'buy into' the need for continuous improvement, and this cannot be achieved in an environment which diminishes self-esteem, confidence and respect.

I have asked an outstanding coaching team, Alan and Sandy Richardson, to expand on the topic of coaching. Their experience as peak performance coaches from the Washington State area will prove to be applicable to teams throughout the United States. I have also enlisted the talents of Dyan Hunter to give you a unique perspective of coaching teams during times of transition. In order to create long-lasting teams, we must expect the best and prepare for the worst. Transitioning is one of these cases. Regardless of the type of transition: dentist retirement, the addition of an associate, the dismissal of key staff members, the expectations and fears of the team rise to a new level. Dyan's expertise will assist you in dealing with these special situations.

Before you proceed into gaining new insights into coaching from Alan and Sandy, let's examine your values as a coach.

Core Coaching Values

To what degree do you believe that the following statements are characteristic of your behavior or performance? Circle the number that you believe applies to you for each statement. Date this evaluation and repeat periodically, initially every three months, using a different colored pen to evaluate your improvement. Have the team complete the companion feedback evaluation to maximize your learning.

Use this as a discussion tool with your team. Find out how you can improve your skills as a coach for the practice.

Answer Key: 1 = very characteristic, 2 = moderately characteristic, 3 = somewhat characteristic, 4 = moderately uncharacteristic, 5 = very uncharacteristic.

1st evaluation _____(date) **Feedback from Team** ___yes ___no
2nd evaluation_____(date) **Feedback from Team** ___yes ___no
3rd evaluation_____(date) **Feedback from Team** ___yes ___no

	High				**Low**

In relationships with my team:

1. I show them I believe that they have a desire to be
   fully competent in their jobs. 1   2   3   4   5

2. I give them the chance to demonstrate competence.
       1   2   3   4   5

3. I encourage them to take on increasingly
   challenging tasks.   1   2   3   4   5

4. I make minimal use of controls.
       1   2   3   4   5

5. I am quick to express appreciation for their efforts
   in a variety of ways.   1   2   3   4   5

6. I allow them to correct their own mistakes and use them
   as learning experiences.   1   2   3   4   5

7. I make sure their work is as interesting and challenging
   as I can make it.   1   2   3   4   5

8. I am available to talk with them about improving
   their performance.   1   2   3   4   5

9. I make it easy for them to tell me if they don't know
   how to do something.   1   2   3   4   5

10. I often initiate conversations to help them perform
    at their top potential.   1   2   3   4   5

Core Coaching Values
Team Feedback

This evaluation can be used for any member of the team that requests feedback on their coaching skills. This is particularly helpful for the doctors, office managers, department heads, and team leaders. To ensure accurate feedback, have each team member complete this and average the score for each question.

Name of the person I am evaluating: _____.

To what degree do you believe that the following statements are characteristic of the person about whom you are completing this questionnaire? Circle the number that you believe applies to that person for each statement.

Answer Key: 1 = very characteristic, 2 = moderately characteristic, 3 = somewhat characteristic, 4 = moderately uncharacteristic, 5 = very uncharacteristic.

	High				**Low**

In relationships with coworkers and team members:

1. Shows coworkers that he/she wants to be fully competent in their jobs.   1   2   3   4   5

2. Gives coworkers the chance to demonstrate their competence.   1   2   3   4   5

3. Encourages coworkers to take on increasingly challenging tasks.   1   2   3   4   5

4. Makes minimal use of controls to manage coworkers performance.   1   2   3   4   5

5. Is quick to express appreciation for coworkers good work.   1   2   3   4   5

6. Gives coworkers opportunity to improve when they make mistakes.   1   2   3   4   5

7. Makes sure work of coworkers is interesting and challenging.   1   2   3   4   5

8. Is easily available to talk about
improving performance.   1   2   3   4   5

9. Makes it easy for coworkers to tell him/her if they don't
know how to do something.   1   2   3   4   5

10. Often initiates conversations to help coworkers perform
at their top potential.   1   2   3   4   5

© 1996 McGraw-Hill, Dennis Kinlaw, <u>ASTD Trainer's Sourcebook: Coaching,</u>
reprinted with permission.

Words of Wisdom

[Coach] each team member to grow emotionally and clinically and to be the best they can be!

DR. JEFF PRILUCK
Dunwoody, GA

After team discussion, we make necessary changes and use them to our advantage. We support one another by complimenting each other and by keeping our agreements.

DR. EUGENE MARKOWSKI
Suffield, CT

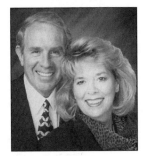

Chapter Twelve

Turn on the 'High Speed':
Coaching High Performance Teams

Alan and Sandy Richardson

"Obstacles are those frightful things you see when you take your eyes off the goal." — HANNAH MOORE

By definition, a high performance team is one that has blended together two primary components — the Achievement Component and the Relationship Component. In the Achievement Component, the team is very clear about and committed to its vision, shared goals, tasks and common interests. In the Relationship Component, members of the team have caring, loving relationships within the team, exhibiting strong evidence of trust, respect, and support — yet hold each other accountable to their high standard. The leader of a high performance team must understand the balance necessary between the two components. The role of the Coach is to review and guide the performance of the team and to ensure the balance between the Achievement and Relationship Components.

Let's look at the characteristics of these components.

The Achievement Component

High performance team members love what they do. They pour their hearts into their work. Doing what you love creates energy and a contagious positive attitude. In all of her interviews, Bonnie Blair, speed skater (gold medal Olympic winner) emphasizes, *"I love to skate!"* High performance teams look for joy in their work because those who are their best at what they do realize that joy lies in working.

High performance team members embrace the goals of the team, always challenging themselves and each other to do better. Goals are regularly established and revised based upon performance. With history as a basis, and the best of companies as models, goals are set from all parameters of the practice from production for each provider and operatory to marketing and staffing levels.

Goals are meaningless unless results are measured, in detail, and in relation to the goals. Monitoring systems, preferably computerized, allow the team on a daily, weekly, and monthly basis to analyze results, take action to correct or enhance results, and celebrate. The individuals who set the goals are accountable to measure, report, and take corrective action. They continually adjust their activities to meet the goals and are highly flexible in the variety and nature of their approaches. The key word here is "ownership." High performance teams declare ownership of all results.

As each new goal is achieved, another one has already been set. The team realizes they are on a journey (some even aspire to being on a pilgrimage) that has no end. They celebrate each outcome as part of the process. The team has certainty in its success, so in order to prevent the fading of focus, interest, and commitment, variety is created. Variety on a daily basis is accomplished by celebrating every possible success and recognizing, as a team, that individual effort is what contributes to the whole. Therefore, the team stays focused on ways to reward and celebrate. A celebration can be as simple as the clinical team ending the day with a group hug or high five for the scheduler. Regardless, celebrations are motivational demonstrations that the more you give, the more you receive. And so, giving becomes a natural part of their culture.

They focus on making the future better than the present. Peak performance coach, Anthony Robbins, in his C.A.N.I.!® model so elegantly states, "Without Continuous and Never Ending Improvement, life becomes jaded and boring. One of our greatest human needs is growth. It is important to continually work to find a better way." The team, particularly the leader, must create an environment where risk is encouraged and failure is regarded as a learning process. A team, whose theme is 'How can we do it even better?' has the potential of moving forward.

They embrace "help." Eager to model others and thriving on learning better ways of doing things, they investigate and research new products, materials, and equipment and are enthusiastic about investments in continuing education. The team knows that by providing their patients the best that their profession has to offer, in terms of procedures, skill, and technology, that growth and profitability are inevitable.

They are excited about creating wealth for themselves and the doctor and have an expectation that high performance deserves high rewards in terms of salary, benefits, and bonuses. The team actively works with the doctor and advisors on how best to invest and manage financial resources so that members can attain a point of financial certainty they so justly deserve.

They do not have, nor can they imagine, an "hourly mentality." They will do 'whatever it takes' to care for their patients and each other even if it means that, on occasion, they have a short lunch or a late day. These high performance teams are unconditional; thus, their work is not a job, but a career. They are clear that if the practice is not functioning smoothly, then they are the ones who can take the necessary corrective action. As colleague, Dick Vessels says, "There are three kinds of people in the world — Winners, Whiners and the Walking Dead." A high performance team is very clear that whining gets nothing, whereas winning gets everything.

They are committed to supporting the achievement and relationship components with weekly staff meetings, knowing the time invested is priceless. They believe that meetings must be positive and productive — providing the platforms to discuss corrections and improvements. These meetings also offer the opportunities to recommit to vision, goals, and support for the team.

They also know that without 'SOOT,' 'SOT,' and 'GOOT,' they cannot sustain high performance on a long term basis. These acronyms are a fun way of coaching time elements throughout the day.

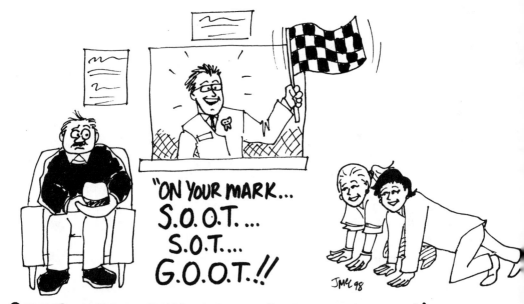

SOOT — is Starting Out On Time. When you begin late, you often end late. When the appointment time is scheduled for 8:00 a.m., this means that the patient is seated at 8:00 a.m.. If a staff member or a doctor is unclear about this, then a team conversation and agreement must take place.

SOT — Staying On Time. Staying on time is the key to reducing stress and chaos for everyone. Time has become an increasingly precious commodity. A contract was established between the patient and the team when the scheduler and the patient agreed upon the appointment time. It is a breach of that contract to run late. Should procedures overrun scheduled times on a regular basis, then they must be re-timed, discussed, and evaluated for clearer scheduling guidelines. If patients are forced to wait more than a few minutes beyond their appointment times, an elegant, honest explanation must be given. The days of unnecessary waiting, are long over… especially in an arena including elective services where the patient has many choices.

GOOT — Getting Out On Time. Getting out on time is a must for every single member of the team. It is an unending source of amazement to this writer that many practices routinely run late, that is, team members working fifteen to twenty minutes after the last patient departed. It is very possible to have it all — high production, happy patients, quality work, enthusiastic team and getting out on time.

A High Performance Team insists on "Morning Huddles" because they know that preparation creates the day… the win, and creates the best environment for their patients. Each day is viewed as a new challenge and an opportunity to do their best. With this focus first thing in the morning, individuals and teams win more frequently because they set themselves up to win. Anything less than this is not an option.

A High Performance Team also insists on an "Evening Huddle" to review the performance of the day and to acknowledge each other for the team effort. Acknowledging great plays of the day stimulates feeling good about accomplishments, reinforcement of the plan, and creates the energy to return the next day and perform at an even higher standard.

They are very clear that the source of their success demands constant focus on the four major components of the "Practice Wheel."

Practice Wellness Wheel

Practice Wellness Wheel

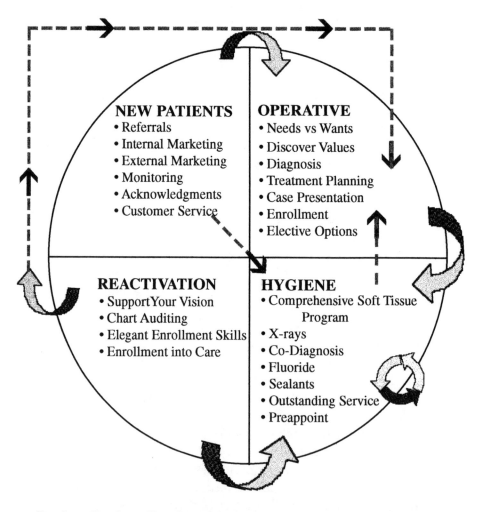

NEW PATIENTS
- Referrals
- Internal Marketing
- External Marketing
- Monitoring
- Acknowledgments
- Customer Service

OPERATIVE
- Needs vs Wants
- Discover Values
- Diagnosis
- Treatment Planning
- Case Presentation
- Enrollment
- Elective Options

REACTIVATION
- SupportYour Vision
- Chart Auditing
- Elegant Enrollment Skills
- Enrollment into Care

HYGIENE
- Comprehensive Soft Tissue
   Program
- X-rays
- Co-Diagnosis
- Fluoride
- Sealants
- Outstanding Service
- Preappoint

**Back to Basics: Continual focus on these four primary areas
ensures great patient care and outstanding success.**

MUSTS: *A willing team committed to C.A.N.I.!®, shared vision, focus, code
of conduct, outstanding relationships, impeccable charting and the integrity
of all communications.*

New Patients — Market continuously, both internally and externally. Internally, the team is clear that within the practice they must ensure that their patients become and remain "Raving Fans" who will refer the majority of new patients. External marketing is a continuum. Daily, the team must have a plan to keep the public informed about their office and incredible services.

Pre-appoint — In a general practice, they make sure no patient departs without an appointment, either in hygiene or operative. The goal is to have every patient of record with an appointment. Pre-appointing takes a proactive team whose pre-appointing goal is in the high 90 percentile. A dental business does not need thousands of files to have a million dollar plus practice. It is easily achievable with twelve hundred patient files. In a specialty practice, all patients are appointed for follow-up, indicative for each specialty.

Reactivation — They review files regularly to ensure that no one has "slipped between the cracks" and follow through with phone contact. The goal for every call is to establish a relationship of trust so that the patient will schedule an appointment to follow through on necessary care.

Diagnosis, Treatment Planning, and Case Presentation — Each member of a high performance team — from administration to the clinical team — is thoroughly familiar with all procedures to better educate and encourage patients regarding oral care opportunities. This is about patients making better choices and allocating resources to meet those choices. If insurance can help, so much the better.

A high performance team is an enrollment machine. It assists patients in sorting through the objections to treatment, making use of high tech tools such as intra-oral cameras, imaging systems, digital radiography, light pen computerization, and basic organization and preparation. Once the patient is informed and takes ownership and responsibility of his teeth and has the desire for improvement, enrollment is largely complete.

A high performance team has FUN!

The Relationship Component

The Relationship Component presents a most challenging paradox… how to maintain close, loving, respectful, supportive empathic relationships while at the same time holding each other to high performance standards on a continual basis. It's imperative that the team knows how to make necessary corrections without "going out of relationship." Being focused on team relationship challenges distracts the focus from the most important person in the practice — the patient.

Managing the Relationship Paradox while keeping the high performance team intact, demands:

Vision, Purpose, Mission Statement — the team must create, be clear, understand, and be committed to their vision.

Agreements or Code of Conduct — through workshops, the team creates agreements that generate a safe work environment, yet supports and assists team members who "lose their way."

Communication Skills — The team works hard on developing elegant, effective, appropriate communication skills in order to maintain high performance.

Coaching

To be an outstanding coach, the following factors must be in place:

Be clear about the characteristics for your team. Take time to think about these and write them down, study them — being specific with your definitions. Include how you want them to act, look, relate, and, most especially, perform. With this clear image, you will coach with ease.

Communicate your expectations. Your team will give you what you need when they clearly understand your expectations.

Clarify responsibilities and roles. Everyone must know his/her job description and each description always includes: "whatever else I can do to support my team."

Create clarity regarding the integrity of the entire team. Individuals have equal accountability and value. Winning or losing is a team effort.

Perhaps you are thinking, "What happens when I have one or more persons on the team who excel, who are always out in front, who are my leaders?" It is a fact that some people are destined to be leaders and will outperform others; nevertheless, it is important to coach those people to integrate their leadership so that the team remains united. Ultimately, star performers should promote team spirit by cheering others' contributions

Be willing for the team to make mistakes. When a team knows there will be no condemnation for errors, they will take productive risks. Thus, believing that there are no failures, but only learning experiences, the team is then free to learn from all experiences. A high performance coach will address these by applauding the success and coaching the errors. When errors occur, the question to ask is: "What do you believe needs to happen to get a *better* result?"

Coaching high performers requires "setting the example." As the coach, you must always be willing to do what you expect from others. The goal is to *lead the team*, rather than *manage the staff*. When the team knows that the coach is willing to lead, by example, they become more willing to commit and recommit.

Use the power of questions to coach your team. Avoid telling, as this puts people on the defensive. Instead, when challenges occur, ask great questions, such as:

- Tell me, what could have occurred differently to produce a better result?
- What would it take right now, for your frustration to diminish?
- In supporting others, we increase our own fulfillment.
- Who could you support today?
- If this (situation) occurs in the future, how can we be better prepared?

As the leader and coach, your goal is to focus on the continued refinement of the team; therefore, your practice will always be in a state of growth, and you will be constantly seeking new talent. When looking to add to the team, be clear on the qualities and skills you are seeking. Look for people who love life, are willing to learn and grow, have positive attitudes, and are enthusiastic about the possibility of having a place on your team. When interviewing, you must leave no doubt about the code of conduct and standards that are requirements on the team, sharing philosophy, values and vision in detail.

Congratulations on your commitment to be the best coach for your team and best wishes to you and your team for a fulfilled journey.

High Performance Teams

The Achievement Component

In a workshop team environment rate yourselves from one to five (five being the highest) on the following:

☐ The team *cooperatively* sets goals and constantly challenges each other.

☐ The team *enthusiastically* measures and monitors all aspects of the results.

☐ The team continually takes action to achieve the goals by *adjusting its approach*.

☐ The team *continually* focuses on making the future better than the present, C.A.N.I.!®

☐ The team loves continuing education and asking for help.

☐ The team insists on problem solving by brainstorming/masterminding.

☐ The team is excited about creating wealth for themselves and the doctor and believe that high performance deserves high rewards.

☐ The team will do whatever it takes to take care of its patients and each other even if it means a short lunch or an occasional late day.

☐ The team starts each day on time.

☐ The team stays on time.

☐ The team ends each day on time.

☐ The team holds weekly staff meetings that are productive and fun.

☐ The team loves Morning Huddles and would not miss them.

☐ The team loves Evening Huddles to review the day and acknowledge each other.

☐ The team pre-appoints in the 90 percentile.

☐ The team chart audits the total patient base at least every six months.

☐ The team is excellent at diagnosis, treatment planning, case presentation and enrollment.

The Relationship Component

Balancing the Achievement Component with the Relationship Component... how to get great results, coach each other, and stay in relationship.

- ❑ The team is committed to a clear simple (shared) vision.
- ❑ The team has agreements *solidly* in place and fully supports them.
- ❑ The team *continually* works to develop elegant, effective communication skills.
- ❑ The team is committed to a Hospitality Culture... approachable at all times.
- ❑ The team is open to new ideas.
- ❑ The team is open and willing to do the little things that make the big differences and will hold the other members of the team to the same standard.

Alan & Sandy Richardson

Alan brings to the business of dentistry, a refreshing, stimulating perspective based on more than 30 years experience in heavy industry and business management. As a Chairman and CEO of public companies and having lived and worked in many parts of the world, his insightful knowledge and experience adds a dimension unique to the field of dentistry… a leader of large teams worldwide. Born in England and educated at King's College, University of London and the Imperial College of Science and Technology in London, his broad international experience adds vitality and energy to everything he does. In addition to operating a large dental consulting business in the Northwest United States, Alan is Executive Director of Fortune Practice Management® a nationwide healthcare consulting company. He is also CEO of Future Life*trends,* Inc., a company focused on enriching the quality of relationships and human communication.

Sandy brings to her profession, a joy and loving presence that affect all whom she meets. Her lecturing, coaching, and seminar leadership create within her participants, a desire to be better at everything they do. Specializing in enriching the human spirit, she has proven to be an example of what is possible. In addition to being President of Fortune Practice Management Northwest, she is the founder and President of Future Life*trends,* Inc., a company with wide-ranging services including Dental Careers Institute, a dental assisting and business administration school and Power of 2 — a subsidiary company dedicated to enriching relationships between the sexes, both professionally and personally. Sandy has extensive experience in banking and management, including Trust Management for a large Midwest banking corporation, marketing for the Federal Reserve Bank System and Foundation Director for Shodair Children's Hospital — Montana.

This dynamic coaching and consulting team can be contacted by phone (888) 495-3623 (4-XLENCE) Fax: (509) 456-8421 or E-mail: Salan2@aol.com

Words of Wisdom 🦷

Team members never take advantage of other team members.
DR. BRIAN HART
Mukilteo, WA

Each of us understands that each appointment, each patient, each procedure requires the effort of each team member. If we are to provide the highest quality of care to our patients, we each have our roles within the team, and understand that our ideas and our actions are a part of the whole.
DR. JOHN T. BLACK, JR.
Pontotoc, MS

As a TEAM, we recognize and model each other's strengths — rather than as an OFFICE, where we (would) dwell on each other's weaknesses.
DR. MATTHEW J. SADLER
Gig Harbor, WA

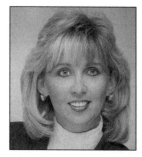

Chapter Thirteen

Your 'Crowning' Achievement: Coaching Your Team Through Transition

Dyan Hunter

"Things do not change, we change." — Henry David Thoreau

Practice transition ranges in scope from restructuring management systems, to incorporating associates or partners into the practice, to the retirement or sale of the lead dentist's interest in the practice. Rather than sharing the horror stories of unsuccessful practice transitions, let's focus on success strategies, which prevent them. This chapter is designed to reinforce and polish the tools that you have already learned in this book. You'll discover that transition (or change) doesn't have to be a fearsome prospect.

Mention the word change and most people shake in their boots. Yet can you imagine your life or practice without change? Without changes, dentists would have little to hope for, plan for, or look forward to.

Change is the creative energy in the life of any dental practice — the source of all learning and growth. As we guide our practices through the transition cycle or face the unexpected (such as disability or death), we have to respond in new ways. And as we change, we learn something new about ourselves as leaders.

A few years ago, we planned a retreat for practices in various stages of our management program. Our goal was to framework a weekend filled with unique challenges for each doctor and team. The itinerary featured white water rafting. Upon gathering at the river, our group of four dentists, 12 staff members, two consultants, and four rafts, was surprised with only three river guides! It was agreed that the experienced rafters — which interestingly consisted of all the doctors and consultants — would occupy the fourth raft.

We devised a plan for these "experienced rafters" to share leadership. It was harmonious in theory, however, as our voyage progressed, so did our frustration. Taking turns at the helm, we exhibited varying leadership styles, none of which proved satisfactory to the entire group. By the end of our adventure, our vision of shared leadership seemed a fairy tale. Meanwhile, the staff was celebrating and sharing stories of victory. Obviously their experience had been much more fulfilling. Our group of "experts" had fallen victim to change and was unguided by a leader's vision.

Transition, or change, is an inevitable and desirable part of practicing dentistry. The real question is: How much direction will you give to the transitions in your practice? Will you be a victim or become a visionary? In order to direct transition, we must first understand it.

Perhaps Max De Pree, author of <u>Leadership Jazz</u> and <u>Leading Without Power</u>, defined transition best. He said:

"For me the idea of transition is one of the most significant ideas that we should be reflecting on today. Transition is a matter and a process of becoming. Transition is a great deal more than change. It's a growing, and a maturing, and an understanding and wisdom-gaining process. Transition gives us the opportunity to rise above polarization. Transition is a marvelous polishing of our intellectual, spiritual and emotional faculties. It's a process of learning who we are. And it's an opportunity to renew our dreams and refresh our calling. Even if we don't experience transition every day, we must surely prepare ourselves for it."

Unlike past years, today's dental practice owner can often look forward to the eventual sale of his or her business. However, with the changing trends in dentistry, it is difficult to know exactly the "right" time to sell. Regardless, practice transitions require effective, dynamic leadership.

In order to make choices for a truly satisfying and fulfilling practice life cycle, you must first determine your values. [To determine what's important to you during times of transition, reread Chapter Two by Nate Booth and repeat the exercises.] Remember the Values and Sparks questions explained by Nate? Ask yourself, "What's most important to me in the lifeline of my practice (Desired Emotional Value)? What has to happen in order for me to feel (Value)?" Also ask "What's most important to me as the coach for my team during times of transition (Desired Emotional Value)? What has to happen in order for me to feel (Value)?" Now aim your practice lifeline in those directions.

A few years ago, I worked with Dr. "W," a young dentist who planned early for the eventual sale of his practice and aimed his practice lifeline in that direction. His experience of the process is definitely worth sharing.

Although Dr. W enjoyed dentistry, he knew early in his career that he wanted to pursue other options as well. After purchasing an existing practice and working successfully through the transition of ownership, Dr. W needed a comprehensive transition plan.

Employed to design and develop his plan, I was impressed with his planning and focus. Together we developed a quite specific, 7-year plan to support him, his vision, and his leadership skills.

Over the next few years we spent hours in leadership coaching and the planning paid off. He was a dedicated student, willing to spend the time to reach his goals. He quickly gained the respect and admiration of his staff as they experienced his growth in leadership.

As Dr. W grew, so did his practice. In fact, the practice soon outgrew the level of capabilities of some initial staff members. Faced with this newfound growth, Dr. W had to make some difficult decisions. As he carefully evaluated which staff members he would continue to coach and lead, he determined that he would need to change his team roster. After hours of role-playing and perfecting his communication skills, Dr. W handled the situation with skill and confidence, which enhanced his credibility with the entire staff. He assisted the former staff members in finding other employment, while his relationship with the remaining staff provided the support to press on toward his goals.

In year five of his plan, he began to position the practice for a future sale. By this time he had developed a highly skilled team of dental

158 ☺ FUNdamentals™ of Outstanding Dental Teams

professionals who also became leaders in the practice. Rather than keeping his future plans of the practice sale secret, he empowered them to help. With no immediate need to sell, he invested the time and energy in his vision, openly answering questions and assuring the staff of their job security.

Energized and excited to help, the staff spent a year getting the practice in immaculate order. All systems were reviewed; financial arrangements were fine-tuned; scheduling was improved; and treatment acceptance was at an all-time high.

During the last two years of Dr. W's practice, the numbers reflected the most profitable years ever! In year seven, Dr. W was ready to sell the practice. With no need to "hide" potential buyers, he opened his doors to interested candidates. Buyer candidates were so impressed with being able to discuss the practice with the staff, review the systems, and evaluate the numbers that Dr. W had four full-price offers on the table within 30 days of listing.

Dr. W also involved the staff in his choice of a purchaser. By inviting their input, he also began the positive transition for the buyer-dentist. Prior to announcing his choice, we drafted a transition letter to patients to insure patient retention. The closing went well. The staff was rewarded for their efforts with a good-bye bonus, a weekend at the Ritz-Carlton, and a transfer of employment to the new owner-dentist.

Dr. W spent the next year on a round-the-world trip providing volunteer dentistry to third-world countries. He later became licensed in other states and now enjoys dentistry in many ways. He has developed a successful business as a temporary-dentist. With his extensive training, skills, and accomplishments, he has gained the respect of practicing dentists during times of disability, extended continuing education courses, and vacations. Having successfully sold his practice at the age of 38, he is busier now than ever.

What made Dr. W's experience so successful? What difference in leadership style, ability and maturity did Dr. W possess?

Successfully guiding your practice through the transition life cycle requires forwardthinking. Clarifying your values and acknowledging your leadership challenges early in the game is the first step. Being actively involved and listening to others supplies you with additional information. Careful examination and refinement of your leadership qualities will make your foundation stronger.

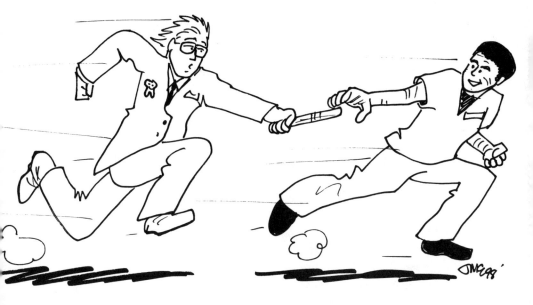

PLANNING CREATES SMOOTH TRANSITIONS!

Helpful Hints for Successful Transitions

- Clarify your values. Decide what you really want.
- If purchasing a practice: host a farewell party for the seller-dentist. Invite patients to your new office to say their good-byes.
- During the first six months of a transition, keep changes to a minimum.
- Build in time for the management of a transition. Have regular staff meetings, develop checklists, and appoint key staff members to implement your action plan.
- A large percentage of the value of any practice is based on goodwill. Put the patients first. Understand their needs and listen to their concerns.
- Plan early for the eventual sale of your practice.
- Understand your P&L Statement and know the details of a healthy overhead.
- With the aid of experts in the field, develop an action plan for unlikely or untimely events. Put the action plan in writing, keep it in a safe place and tell your spouse or significant other where it is.
- Have your practice valued by a transition specialist. Don't use "ballpark" estimates to value your practice.
- Decide when it is best to inform the staff of a practice transition. Empower them by keeping them informed and ask for their support. Reward your staff in the process.
- Streamline your office and organize your systems prior to a practice sale or transition.
- Develop communication scripts for the transition of an associate; role-play them with staff.
- Develop a practice transition letter that effectively communicates that the patient is the most important factor in the process.
- Enthusiastically support the transition and show confidence in your successor.
- Once you've sold the practice, LET GO!

Developing a Practice Transition Lifeline

Understanding the flow of the practice transition cycle prepares better leaders. In order to understand the dynamics of this cycle, try putting your practice on the line for a closer look at the changes along the way. We call this process the Practice Transition Life-Line. Let's look at how it works:

Write down eight to 10 major events that best represents changes in your practice since you started. (such as: purchase, hiring associate, building new facility, etc.)

Arrange these chronologically.

List events that have required you to change your leadership style. (For example, hiring/managing larger staff; relocating, hiring an associate, etc.)

Compare these two lists and answer the following questions

Which were the most important changes in your practice lifeline?

What did you learn as a leader during these changes?

Which changes did you direct and what was your leadership style during the process? (example: passive, controlling, motivational, etc.)

What did you do to make these changes happen and how effective were you as a leader?

Gain another perspective by having a long term-employee, accountant, consultant or someone involved in your practice answer the following questions:

1. What changes in leadership have you noticed in me since I began my practice?
2. What changes have you seen in the people and things that are important to me?
3. What changes have you observed in the way I seem to feel about my leadership in the practice?
4. Which of these changes do you think has had the greatest impact?
5. In what ways have I helped to direct these changes?

Look over the responses and answer these questions:
1. How does this person's view of your leadership match yours?
2. Did this person's responses surprise you in any way?

Once you complete this exercise, compare your view with others and complete the following to determine the core lifeline of your practice.

Three qualities I like about who I am as a leader in my practice are:
1._____
2._____
3._____

Two accomplishments in my leadership that I feel good about are:
1._____
2._____

Three times I successfully coached my team during transition were:
1._____
2._____
3._____

Draw from these distinctions and model your past success to follow your practice lifeline into a successful future.

Dyan Hunter

Dyan Hunter, practice management consultant, lecturer and writer, enjoys coaching and training doctors and their staff in the ever-changing world of practice transitions.

With a degree in Visual Communications and Marketing combined with over eight years in the corporate banking industry, she brings new insight to leaders in dentistry. Dyan began her career in dentistry as a consultant with the Pride Institute of San Francisco, CA and later founded *The Learning Center for Practice Enhancement Services* in Atlanta, GA. She has provided dentists and staff with "hands-on" training and coaching for the past 10 years, specializing in transition management.

In 1997, Dyan, along with colleagues Brenda Hunt and Malcolm H. Kerstein, D.D.S., personal-growth coaches and counselors, formed *The Ballastone Group*, a values-based organization focusing on leadership and relationship advancement coaching for successful entrepreneurs in dentistry. Their 3-day dentist/spouse workshop entitled *The Power of Authenticity*, designed for values clarification and life-change management is a must for principle-centered leaders in dentistry.

For additional information or to order the tape series *Communication Skills — Survival Tools for Practice Transitions* contact Dyan Hunter, The Ballastone Group (813) 593-2163.

Words of Wisdom

Promoting team in our office starts with hiring employees with positive attitudes and outstanding communication skills. Also, cross training benefits when others need assistance and individuals are able to appreciate and respect specific job titles.

DR. DEBRA KING
Atlanta, GA

A team's focus and morale may wax and wane from time to time. The difference between short lived highs and long term success stems from having strong team building blocks in place, rather than systems. Essentials such as team agreements, strong communication skills, and above all, a focused and powerful vision are mandatory. A team moving in one direction is unstoppable!!

DR. MICHAEL J. KOCZARSKI
Woodinville, WA

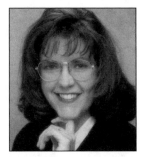

Chapter Fourteen

Holy 'Molar'... This should be FUN? Celebrating, Rewarding, and Motivating your Team

Penny Reed

"That which gets rewarded, gets done." — DR. JOHN MAXWELL

Can you imagine attending a sporting event where there was no way to keep score, no winner? How exciting would that be? How would you know when to cheer? How would you know when to celebrate? We all need a purpose; we need to know the rules; we need to know when to celebrate; and we need to know when we've won! Knowing when you've won the game is one of the greatest challenges that takes place in the business of dentistry.

Which came first, the wins or the fans? Most of the time, the fans don't show up until the team starts winning. *Your fans are quality patients and quality staff members.* As the leader of your team, accept responsibility and instill the winning spirit. As doctors, you must follow the golden rule by treating your staff members and patients with the same appreciation and respect you would like to receive. By giving what you want, you reap a tremendous return on your investment, both emotionally and financially.

Speaking the Language of a Winner

Why is it important to feel you are winning? If you feel as if you are winning and yet don't have the production month you need to have, you won't waste a lot of time worrying about it. Rather, you will ask yourself and your team "What do we need to do to reach our goals next month?" If you feel you are losing and having a less than desirable month, you are likely to feel improvement is impossible and stop trying. Can you imagine a basketball player who, after missing a shot, lies down on the floor and gives up, rather than chasing the rebound?

How do you describe unfortunate incidents or lack of results in your practice and your life? Doctors and staff who give in easily when facing challenges will describe their situations with statements like "We will never be successful in this town," "It's me; I am not a good leader and cannot keep my staff motivated," or "Managed care is going to undermine everything we do." On the other hand, doctors and staff who do not give in easily say "It was just a slow month, we'll bounce back" or "If we refocus on improving the quality of care we deliver and our marketing plan, we can attract the patients we need."

In his book <u>Learned Optimism</u>, Dr. Martin P. Seligman labels the way you describe events in your life as your explanatory style. Dr. Seligman mentions two components of your explanatory style: *permanence* and *pervasiveness.*

Permanence

People who stick with their goals in spite of poor circumstances or undesired results describe their situation as temporary, while those who give up easily will describe their situation as permanent.

It is much more difficult to handle a disappointment using qualifiers such as *always* and *never* to describe your situation. To handle disappointments quickly use words such as *temporary* or *lately*. For example, after a low production month, one doctor might respond "We will never achieve our production goals consistently," a *permanent* description. Another doctor might respond, "Last month was a little rough," making the disappointment seem *temporary*.

Pervasiveness: Specific vs. Universal

Permanence is about the length of time a result will last. The next "P" pervasiveness deals with the dimension of a good or bad experience. People who give *universal* explanations for a negative experience in one area may give up in all areas of their lives. People who give *specific* explanations for a disappointing experience may give up in one area yet remain steady in others. "The only treatment that patients want to have done is what insurance will cover" is a *universal* statement that all patients are the same and would not want optimal treatment. An example of a *specific* statement would be "It seems that this patient may only want to proceed with treatment which insurance will cover." This gives a sense of optimism to case acceptance.

By maintaining a positive attitude and limiting the scope of your disappointments, you encourage the team to adopt empowering beliefs. Speak the language of a winner to motivate your team!

How do you know when you've won? In order to win, you must first have a clear working definition of winning. You must be able to communicate this definition in a way that empowers you to work toward your goals when both good and bad events take place. And you must create a plan to let you and your team know when and how to celebrate your wins.

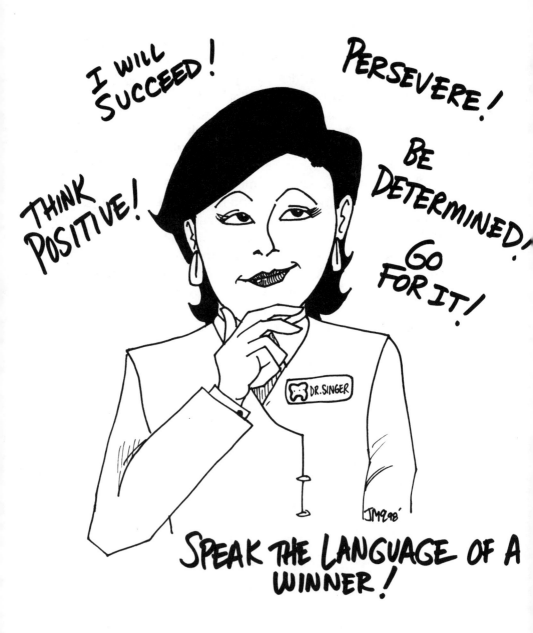

Your Definition of Winning

Ball games have scoreboards; races have winners, so how do you know when you've won in a dental practice? Here are typical replies to this question.

- When we have reached our goals.
- When ALL scheduled patients show up.
- When we get a bonus.
- When we have a full schedule, booked to goal, every day.
- When we have lots of referrals.

How many of the above must happen for you to feel you're winning? All of them? Have you ever seen a baseball game where every batter hit home runs, or where the pitcher only threw strikes? The best players in major league baseball only get a hit 30% of the time and pitchers rarely pitch shutout games, much less throwing all strikes!

The belief seems to be that unless we are "perfect" and reach all of our goals we have failed. We are our own worst enemy! We deny ourselves victory. Where is the motivation to continue to play the game if you will never win? Let's look at an adaptation of a "Rules" exercise from Chapter 16 of <u>Awaken the Giant Within</u> by Anthony Robbins to discover if you have disempowering rules for winning.

You have a disempowering rule for winning if it is almost impossible to meet. When there are too many events that must occur, then winning is so complex that you won't ever experience it.

You have a disempowering rule for winning if something you can't control determines whether you win. For example, if your patients *must always* accept full comprehensive care, or staff *must* exceed their goal everyday, without exception, you definitely have a disempowering rule for winning.

Your rule for winning is disempowering if it gives you only a few opportunities to feel good and many ways to feel bad.

You, and your team, must redesign your definition for winning so that it is achievable on a daily basis. The key is to make it easier to win and harder to lose. Your self-esteem is tied directly to your ability to feel in control of your situation. Remember you are always in control of the way you define and react to your circumstances.

Consider these definitions for winning:

We learned a better way to serve our patients today.
We educated our patients about their dental health.
We were acknowledged for our expertise and gentle care.
We are on target to produce and collect fees needed to meet our financial goals.

Giving Your Team That Winning Feeling

Most dentists are very open to rewarding their teams for jobs well done. When managed appropriately, an incentive plan can be cost effective and produce tremendous emotional and financial benefits in your business. There are four key steps in formulating your rewards plan.

Know your objective. You and your team must have goals. Your incentive program should also be aligned with your mission statement and your business plan for the practice. The best way to do this is to create the top ten targets of your business plan and the top ten ways to reward them.

Create a plan. Be sure that your objectives are clearly defined and that you measure progress. For example, if you have a contest that rewards the staff member who refers the most patients to the practice each month, you need to track the referral sources of all your new patients. You need to let your team know what the incentive will be, for example, a $50 bonus. You also need to be clear about the length of time the program will be in effect — three months, six months, one year, etc.

Establish awards. The most effective way, to stay energized about your staff incentive programs, is to establish a spending plan for your awards. Next decide the different levels and frequency.

In 1001 Ways to Reward Employees, Bob Nelson gives three guidelines for acknowledging staff:
- ❑ The reward should match the staff member's personality and interests
- ❑ The reward should match the achievement
- ❑ The reward should be done in a timely manner and should be specific.

Measure your results. Notice the team's reaction and comments regarding the rewards. Did you notice extra excitement generated from certain awards? Periodically ask your staff what they like best about their reward's program. Also, look at your practice productivity. Has there been a measurable change in production? Are you seeing more new patients? Have you been receiving more compliments from your patients?

Here are some specific ways to reward and praise your staff:

Written acknowledgments are an excellent source and will give long term results. Many times your team may not remember compliments given to them; however, they can keep a letter or note you have given them and feel good every time they read it.

Praise cards*:* Ken Blanchard's live seminar, *Mission Possible: Becoming A World-Class Organization While There Is Still Time,* discusses the importance of understanding that "everyone is your partner." He created a post card, which had printed on one side, "Eagle of The Moment" which he sent to anyone who went the extra mile. Dr. Blanchard would write a personal message describing how this person had made a special contribution and sent these cards to all sorts of people: his staff, helpful airline agents, and president's of corporations.

Develop a praise card, at least 3x5 in size, to acknowledge not only your office team, but also your patients, suppliers, and others who contribute to or are associated with your business.

Personal notes: One of the most heartfelt thank-you's I ever received from an employer was a handwritten note. In the note he thanked me for my hard work and for treating the practice as if it were my own. That note was written almost four years ago, and I still have it. A great point to remember is that rewards and praise are not directly tied to money. Here is a sample letter to use as a guide in giving your staff members written acknowledgment.

Sample Acknowledgment Letter

Dear _____ (be sure to personalize for each staff member)

You are such an important part of my team and my life. I would like to thank you for. . . your willingness to try new things. This is such an important part of our continued growth as a practice.

Believing in my capabilities and me. Thank you for giving me unconditional support and complementing my work.

Your dedication. You have been with me for two years now and I feel as if you are part of my family. Thanks for sticking with me during good times and bad.

Your commitment to our patients. I have so much confidence in you and your abilities. It is so comforting to know that I have you on our team to care for our patients.

Your caring spirit. Thank you for the compassion that you show to our patients and other members of our team. You are a great listener and a wonderful example.

Your honesty and your commitment to open and supportive communication. I really value your integrity.

Your willingness to accept challenges and continuing to add value in our office. You are a valuable team member. Thank you for understanding that we must have a profitable business in order to take care of our patients and ourselves.

I have really enjoyed the past two years. I look forward to many more. I am glad you are on my team.

Thank you!

Dr.'s first name

Other ideas to make personal notes more special:

Mail them to your staff's home address.
Write a thank-you note to your staff's spouses and family letting them know how much you appreciate them in supporting your staff members and their roles in the practice.

Bonus plans: Having an incentive plan where the staff has the opportunity to earn more is vital in having your team "step-up" in the practice. Because there are many variables involved in establishing a bonus plan, be sure and run the numbers to see what will work for your business plan. Two key points to remember when implementing a bonus plan: (1) Base the bonus on collections, not production, and (2) Be sure every staff member has the opportunity to participate in the bonus plan.

Public praise: (p.38 1001 Ways to Reward Employees, Bob Nelson) Take out an ad in your local newspaper every year and acknowledge your team by name for the contribution they make to your practice.

Make rewards and praise a priority. That which is scheduled gets done. In our fast-paced world, most of us live by a calendar or appointment book where we schedule everything that is "important." If you want to make a habit out of giving others the gift of winning, you must schedule it. Create an acknowledgment calendar. Use this calendar to schedule acknowledgments for your patients, staff, and referral sources.

Also, remember to be spontaneous. The rewards and praise that will be remembered as most special will be the rewards that didn't have to be earned. The staff didn't have to meet a quota and it doesn't have to be a birthday or holiday. "Just Because" rewards will have a tremendous impact and let your staff know that they are important to you. Your team needs a pick-me-up every 60 to 90 days. Schedule your "Just Because" awards accordingly.

Knowing what winning is, communicating winning to yourself and your team, and having a system in place that rewards your wins are initial components to coaching your team to success. Remember that winning is a mindset, not a destination. You must train yourself and your team to adopt a winning philosophy to empower you to strive for fulfillment and continual growth in your business.

Creating Your Rules for Winning

Part I
    Have each person create three new definitions for winning that can easily be achieved on a daily basis and are independent of an outside source:

I feel as if I've won when...

_____

_____

I feel as if I've won when...

_____

_____

I feel as if I've won when...

_____

_____

Part II
Have each person share his/her new definitions for winning and make a list of the top five. You now have team rules for winning.

Our Team Rules for Winning:

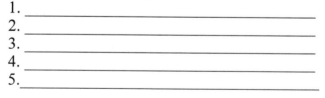

    1. _____

    2. _____

    3. _____

    4. _____

    5. _____

Part III
Transform your team rules for winning into <u>Daily Focus Questions</u>. You will use these questions as a measuring stick for winning. Use open-ended questions as opposed to yes or no questions. The best way to do this is to preface the questions with: "How did we...?" or "In what ways did we...?"

For example, how did we show concern for our patients and deliver quality care today?

1._____
2._____
3._____
4._____
5._____

Part IV

Ask these questions at either the morning huddle or the end of the day debriefing. Use them to empower your team and reinforce good attitudes and behavior.

Penny L. Reed

For nearly a decade, Penny has been empowering businesses to become more productive and profitable. Her comprehensive background in management, leadership, and team building is facilitated by first-hand experience as part of a dynamic health care team.

Ms. Reed earned her BBA in Business Management from Harding University. As a coach and consultant with Fortune Practice Management® — Memphis, Tennessee, Ms. Reed actively assists dental practices in building fulfilling businesses and stable, highly productive teams. For more information, please call (901) 371-9056 or Fax (901) 386-5889, or E-mail FPMMemphis@compuserve.com.

Words of Wisdom 🦷

We celebrate anything that I can think of that involves staff to promote recognition. Employees receive gifts on birthdays and employment anniversaries, which can be enjoyed by staff and patients — such as flowers, balloons, lunches, etc.

DR. RICHARD BERMAN
Thousand Oaks, CA

I try to involve the staff in projects or events outside the practice. [For example, we once had] a limo arrive at 10 a.m., each staff member was given $100 and we went to the shopping mall.

DR. WILLIAM OAKES
New Albany, IN

We do things together. We have an annual Christmas party where all staff members are encouraged to bring their spouses and children. We have an annual (family) trip to our local water park.

DR. BRIDGETT BORRIS
Las Cruces, NM

At staff meetings, each staff member is given a $5.00 bill to award to another in recognition of "above and beyond" behavior. It encourages us to catch each other being good and keeps us aware of how important it is to look for opportunities to help. Praise from peers feels great!

DR. TERRI L. BRUMMITT
San Jose, CA

Schedule a "ghost" day with false appointments and when the staff comes to work, take them water-skiing, or snow mobiling, bungy jumping or something they would really enjoy!

DR. BRET TOBLER
Provo, UT

Recommended Reading List

Awaken the Giant Within, by Anthony Robbins; Summit Books 1991

Built to Last, by James C. Collins and Jerry I. Porras; Harper
  Business 1994

Finding the Magnetic Leader — Moving from Personal Chaos to
  Personal Peace, Nick Nicholas, CSP, and Steve Cohn; Radkin
  Publishing 1997, 800-925-5788

Focus, by Al Reis; Harper Business 1996

Gung Ho!, by Ken Blanchard and Sheldon Bowles; Morrow 1998

Raving Fans, by Ken Blanchard and Sheldon Bowles 1993

The New Leader: Bringing Creative and Innovation to the Workplace,
  by Gregory P. Smith; St. Lucie Press 1996

Resources for Outstanding Teams

Anthony Robbins Companies, 800-445-8183

DCU - Standard Operating Procedures (SOP's) for Dental Practice,
  Marsha Freeman 1996, 800-563-1454

Fortune Practice Management®
  Reference: FUN4U, 800- 628-1052 x 6287

FUNdamentals™ of Outstanding Dental Teams Newsletter by
  Fax: (770) 512-0892

MW Corporation, Skill-Building for Self-Directed Teams,
  914-528-0888

National Dental Network, Video Staff Meetings, 800-803-6786

The Profitable Dentist Newsletter, 800-337-8467

Resource List

A. Paul Bass, III, D.D.S.
101 Ogee Street
Tullahoma, Tn 37388
Phone (800) 687-3393
Fax (931) 455-0522
FPMMIDTN@compuserve.com
Practice Mastery (audio tape series)

Nate Booth, D.D.S.
1183 Calle Christopher
Encinitas, CA 92024
Phone: (800) 917-0008
Fax: (760) 753-1995
nbooth@natebooth.com
Thriving on Change: The Art of Using Change to Your Advantage
The Platinum Touch: How to Give People what They Uniquely Desire

Linda Drevenstedt
5691 Musket Lane
Stone Mountain, GA 30087
Phone: (800) 242-7648
Fax: (770) 414-4523
drevgrp@aol.com

Carol Hacker
209 Cutty Sark Way
Alpharetta, GA 30005
Phone (770) 410-0517
Fax (770) 667-9801
GaonMIND@aol.com
Hiring Top Performers – 350 Great Interview Questions For People
Who Need People.
Cost of Bad Hiring Decisions & How to Avoid Them.
High Cost of Low Morale… and what to do about it.

Dr. Paul Homoly
500 H Clanton Road
Charlotte, NC 28217
Phone: (800) 294-9370
Fax: (704) 522-9961
phomoly@aol.com
Dentists: An Endangered Species

Dyan Hunter
1390 Gulf Blvd., Suite 1204
Clearwater, FL 33767
Phone: (813) 593-2163
Communication Skills — Survival Tools for Practice Transitions (audio)

Cathy Jameson
Rt 1 — 2 miles East, 3 miles North
P.O. Box 488
Davis, OK 73030
Phone: (580) 369-5555
Fax: (580) 369-3352
Great Communication = Great Production
Collect what you Produce

Brenda Kaesler, RDH
1861 Timber Trail
Vista, CA 92083
Phone: (760) 727-4509
Fax: (760) 727-8552
FPMDALLAS@compuserve.com

Linda L. Miles, CMC, CSP
4356 Bonney Road, Suite 2-103
Virginia Beach, VA 23452
Phone: (800) 922-0866
Fax: (757) 498-0290
LLMILES@ix.netcom.com

Vicki McManus, RDH
5579-B Chamblee Dunwoody Road, Suite 207
Atlanta, GA 30338
Phone: (888) 347-4785
Fax: (770) 512-0892
FPMVicki@compuserve.com
FUNdamentals™ of Outstanding Dental Teams

Penny Reed
2566 Sunbury Circle
Memphis, TN 38133
Phone: (901) 371-9056
Fax: (901) 386-5889
FPMMemphis@compuserve.com

Alan & Sandy Richardson
1006 South Carousel Lane
Spokane, WA 99224-2003
Phone: (888) 495-3623
Fax: (509) 456-8421
Salan2@aol.com

Doug Smart
PO Box 768024
Roswell, Ga 30076
Phone: (770) 587-9784
Fax: (770) 587-1050
DougSmart.Seminars@worldnet.att.net
TimeSmart: How Real People Really Get Things Done at Work
TimeSmart: How Real People Really Get Things Done at Home
Reach for the Stars

Index

Ordering Information

To obtain additional copies:

Fax orders: 770-512-0892
E-mail: FPMVicki@compuserve.com
Telephone: 888-347-4785
Mail: Lifetime Learning Center
              5579-B Chamblee Dunwoody Road, Suite 207
              Atlanta, GA 30338

Please send me _____ copies of <u>**FUN**damentals</u>™ <u>of</u>
<u>Outstanding Dental Teams</u>

Quantity Pricing:
    1 - 5 copies @ $21.00 ea.   11 - 25 copies @ $17.00
    6 - 10 copies @ $19.00   26 + copies @ $15.00
                      Total: $_____
GA residents add 7% sales tax: $_____

Add $3.00 for first book and $.75 ea
   additional book for Shipping/Handling $_____

Enclosed is a check or money order payable to
Lifetime Learning Center   TOTAL $_____

For faster delivery — fax credit card orders to 770-512-0892

Please charge my (circle one) MasterCard Visa

_____
Account number   Exp Date

_____
Signature (credit card orders only)

Print your address for shipping:
Name: _____
Address: _____
City, State, Zip: _____
Phone: (_____)_____

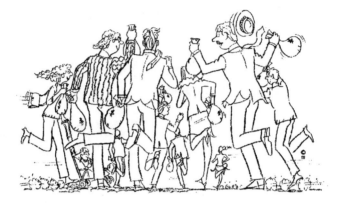

Need a speaker for your next meeting?

Call
Lifetime Learning Center
at 888-347-4785

My Action Ideas: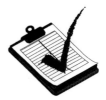

_____

_____

_____

_____

_____

_____

_____

_____

_____

_____

_____

_____

_____

_____

_____

_____

_____

_____

_____

More of My Action Ideas: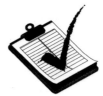

_____

_____

_____

_____

_____

_____

_____

_____

_____

_____

_____

_____

_____

_____

_____

_____

_____

_____